The Dish

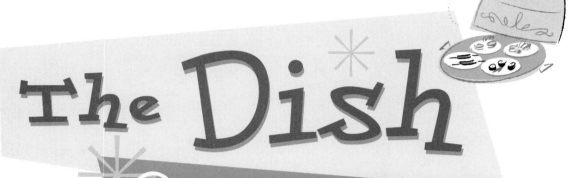

The Dish

On Eating Healthy and Being Fabulous!

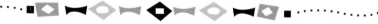

CAROLYN O'NEIL
AND
DENSIE WEBB

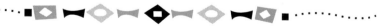

ATRIA BOOKS
New York London Toronto Sydney

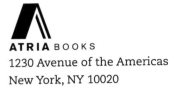

ATRIA BOOKS

1230 Avenue of the Americas
New York, NY 10020

Library of Congress Cataloging-in-Publication Data

O'Neil, Carolyn.
    The dish : on eating healthy and being fabulous / Carolyn O'Neil and Densie Webb.
   —1st Atria Books hardcover ed.
      p. cm.
    ISBN 0-7434-7688-3
      1. Women—Nutrition—Popular works. 2. Women—Health and hygiene—Popular
works. I. Webb, Densie. II. Title.

RA778.O485 2004
613.2—dc22

                                                            2004047699

First Atria Books hardcover edition June 2004

Design by Joel Avirom and Jason Snyder
Design assistant: Meghan Day Healey

10 9 8 7 6 5 4 3 2 1

ATRIA BOOKS is a trademark of Simon & Schuster, Inc.

Manufactured in the United States of America

For information regarding special discounts for bulk purchases,
please contact Simon & Schuster Special Sales at 1-800-456-6798 or
business@simonandschuster.com.

Acknowledgments

The Dish would never have made it to the table without the support of our smart friends and creative colleagues. We'd like to thank our literary agent, Jenny Bent, for believing it was time for a healthy eating book that was fun to read. Big thanks to cool dietitian and cookbook author Liz Weiss, who suggested we call Jenny. Networking at its best! And we can't say enough about the joy of working with the entire team at Simon & Schuster, Atria Books. During our initial tour of publishers we liked them the best and, thankfully, they picked us, too. Our patient and supportive editor, Greer Hendricks, had the wisdom to prod us gently through the writing process and motivate us with praise. Thank you, Greer! Special thanks go to publisher, Judith Curr; editorial director, Tracy Behar; director of publicity, Seale Ballenger, and senior publicist, Brigid Brown.

And we all know that *The Dish* would not have come alive without the uniquely dishy illustrations by artist Laura Coyle. A big thank you to all of our Hip & Healthy Heroines and Gourmet Gurus who lent their behind-the-scenes stories, expertise, and recipes to spice up our pages.

Carolyn Says: Densie, thank you for asking if I would like to write a book with you! My answer was yes and now it's, "Let's do it again!" You are a breeze to work with and when you were yin, I was yang, and vice versa. Huge thanks go to all of my pals who nudged me through the procrastination process of writing a book. Jennifer and Ali, you're next! Ruth, thanks for the original fun idea. Reggie, you kept me focused on the positive. Rhonda, you're a powerful cheerleader. Linda, thank you for taking care of the home front. Mom and Dad, please keep bragging; it really helps. Jack and Katie, thank you for being proud of your mom; I'm proud of you. And just when I thought I'd never get it done, Ann Dunaway became my amazing assistant, organizing everything from research to recipe testing. They say it takes a village, and my town rocks!

Densie Says: First I simply must thank my co-author and fellow Dish Diva, Carolyn O'Neil. She has an amazing amount of energy and a continuous flow of creative juices that we were able to harvest and bottle for *The Dish*. We make an awesome team, Carolyn, if I do say so myself. And I have to give a big hug and a kiss to my significant other, Jacques, whom I married on an impulse years ago and never looked back, and our kids, Ethan and Eliana, who think they're now going to be famous. And I would be remiss if I didn't thank our dog, Brooklyn, who kept me company, lo those many hours, while I was researching and writing the book. I couldn't have done it without their support.

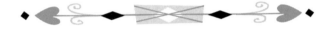

Acknowledgments

Contents

Deep Dish

Welcome to *The Dish on Eating Healthy and Being Fabulous!* a girlfriend's guide to eating out, eating in, entertaining, and traveling. This book was born to bring you fresh advice on making healthier food choices without giving up your right to be fabulous. And, in our world, that doesn't mean staying home with a fridge full of celery and a closet full of rice cakes. *Mais non!* We believe that the more you know about nutrition, the *more* you can eat. So, get ready to dig in to our book full of festive ideas and delicious foods to help you make the best choices at supermarkets, restaurants, airports, and even potential trouble spots like fast-food places and convenience stores. Today's modern, multitasking women are on the move and often need to live off the land, grabbing snacks and meals where and when they can. This book aims to be a gourmet guide, providing women with calorie-saving solutions for all kinds of mealtime situations without sacrificing what matters most—taste!

Written by us—Carolyn and Densie—two registered dietitians who love to eat, we believe that even the most desirable delicacies, from chocolate truffles to chili cheese dip, *can* be part of an overall healthy diet, as long as you only *accessorize* with the rich and fluffy stuff. Just go easy, gal. Everyone knows that overdoing the belts, baubles, bangles, and beads can ruin an outfit. The same goes for designing your dinnertime.

Who needs *The Dish*? Maybe you relate to the single Sex-and-the-City types or a modern mom à la Katie Couric; or you see yourself more as a full-of-life Star Jones or a sleek and timeless Lauren Hutton. No matter. We wanted *The Dish* to be the very first diet book aimed at glamour girls of all ages and sizes. So, don't look here for a long list of what *not* to eat or a strict deprivation diet. Instead, we'd rather share a new way of thinking about food choices, so that you can adapt healthy eating to your personal style and tastes. It's a customized approach that fits you and your lifestyle. Don't like fish? Don't eat it. Gotta have cream in your coffee? Fine. Research shows that if personal preferences are a priority, healthy eating habits can become more than a diet; they become a lifestyle.

But even though we do say *yes* to everything from martinis to mocha fudge, *The Dish* respects the rule that calories in must not exceed calories out. So, get ready to learn some powerful food and fitness strategies to add energy to your days, while subtracting inches from your derriere. Most important, we know that diets don't have to be dull and boring, and neither does a diet book. So, we're not going to dwell on the latest research findings, unless they pass our test, which demands, "Don't tell me what's new, tell me what's true!" And we won't bore you with a lot of scientific mumbo jumbo or diet boot camp lectures. Think of it as nutrition aptitude meets a new diet attitude, full of modern taste and style. Sure, nutrition used to be nerdy, but now it's hip and healthy. Just like you! Here's a sneak preview of what's in store.

☀ Let's Make Healthy Eating Fun and Stylish

You know that fashionable friend who always seems to order the lightest, yet best-tasting dish from the menu? Or that pal who's just as busy as you, but can throw a dinner party almost every weekend and still slip into a little black dress? This book will show *you* how to be like them. There's no need to deprive yourself with dry broiled fish when you can savor grilled salmon brushed with olive oil scented with lemon and dill. And yes, you can entertain guests when you're eating lighter; chances are they'll love you even more for putting on a spread of colorful fresh foods. And here's the bonus! A lifestyle of healthy eating habits not only pays off by controlling the pounds, good nutrition adds bounce to your step, glow to your skin, and shine to your hair. It's the ultimate health and beauty treatment.

☀ Let's Be Healthy by Eating More, Not Less

There's a refreshing change afoot (with a perfect pedicure, of course). Instead of self-deprivation and a long list of foods to avoid, we spin the wheel the other way and offer a long overdue food philosophy that really works. . . . *Eating more!* Let's banish starvation diets that backfire, boring meal plans, and bossy food restrictions. Simply said, strict diets don't cut it. Research shows that such an "all-or-nothing attitude" often leads to overeating, because it makes you feel like you've already blown it if even a single forbidden food passes your lips. The twisted logic then becomes—why not go all the way?

Say good-bye to negative nutrition and hello to newfound freedom, when you choose foods based on what they *add* to your life and health. So, rather than blaming foods for all your ills and bulges, it's time to set a new table with the delicious and nutritious concept of eating *more* foods that are good for you in so many ways. We'll tell you which foods can help power you with energy, control your appetite, boost your immune system, fight disease, and yes, offer a winning edge in weight control. Let's eat!

Let's Fit Healthy Eating into a Hectic Life

Breakfast may be the most important meal of the day, but who has time to garnish a cantaloupe and fold mushrooms into an egg white omelet? Almost no one, unless it's the weekend. That's why *The Dish* presents healthy eating plans that fit into your modern-day, fast-track mode. Rather than the typical menus that dictate what you should eat on Monday, Tuesday, and Wednesday, etc., *The Dish* offers meal solutions in chapter 10 that reflect real women in real-life situations, just trying to eat as healthy as they can, when and where they can. Some days are tougher than others. So we offer suggestions for the times you have to eat on the run or just can't say no to ice cream. It happens! Today's a travel day? We'll help you cope with airport food courts and lousy in-flight food. Have to eat at a restaurant someone else picked? We'll help you navigate any menu. The secret to eating healthier in the fast lane is having a plan. We'll show you how, with simple tips. Grab the car keys!

Let's Learn What Works

Finally, *The Dish* is all about making choices. At lunch should you order the grilled chicken salad or the chicken-salad sandwich? At Happy Hour, what'll it be—a strawberry daiquiri, Chardonnay, or vodka and tonic? Dessert tonight? Should you choose the fresh berries and frozen yogurt or a slice of peach cobbler shared with a friend? To help you learn how to cut calories where they count and maximize flavor and fun when you want to, we dish up easy-to-cook recipes, tips, and techniques from top chefs we call our Gourmet Gurus. To show you what works for other chic women, we profile our Hip & Healthy Heroines, who share their tried and true secrets to slimming success. We'll also dish out ideas for looking great when you still have those five, ten, fifteen, or even more pounds left to lose, plus our own tales from the trenches. We'll tell you how you can enjoy everything from French fries to foie gras, tuna to tenderloin, seltzer to champagne, bottled water to wine, while you live a vibrant, happy life. Also sprinkled throughout the book's pages, you'll find special boxed items filled with all kinds of fun stuff about food. So, read on in any order you choose. Begin by turning the page or start with a few drinks (chapter 6) or go straight to cheating (chapter 8). We just hope you have as much fun reading these pages as we did writing them. Now, let's learn to live it up, be healthy, and look fabulous!

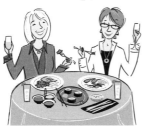

Dish Divas,
Carolyn and Densie
www.dishdivas.com

The Dish

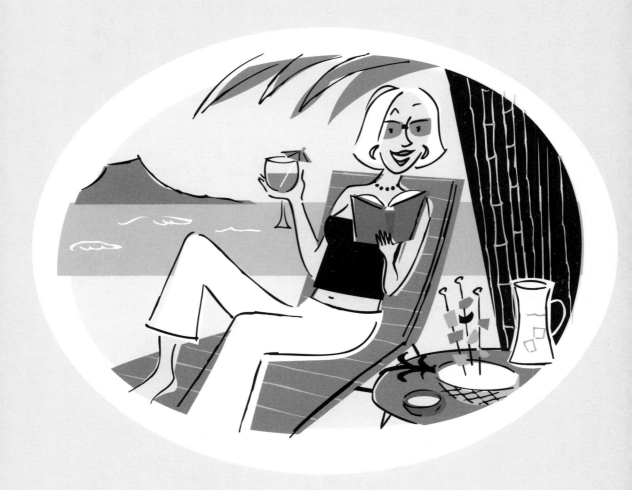

1 The Dish on Your Diet

Welcome to the club, girl! You're about to become one of us now—that elite but growing group of smart, stylish women who have learned that the more you know, the more you can eat. That fact has been, up to now, a well-kept secret. But we see no reason to keep it that way any longer. You may have seen others who wine and dine while staying fit and trim and wondered, "How *do* they do it!" Well, we would like to answer that question for you. Because once the truth is revealed, it will set you free. Free to be a healthier, happier, more sane and more satisfied you. And, oh yes, there's that little matter of your weight. By following our advice, you'll be able to control your weight with less of the confusion, punishment, and emotional drama that usually go hand-in-hand with traditional "dieting." This is the real deal. There's no magic formula here, only the magic that lies in telling the truth. And the truth about eating is simpler and easier than you think. But more about that later.

Before we fill you in on the details about what you need to know so you can eat more, we'd like you to put yourself to the test. Take our *Dish Diet Quiz* to help you pinpoint the weakest links in your soon-to-be new way of looking at food. (No matter how committed you may be, we all have buttons that, once pushed, are hard to turn off.) We want you to be brutally honest with yourself. What sets off your irreversible eating launch sequence—emotions, circumstances, habit? What are your typical triggers—10 A.M. coffee break, after-work drinks, dates, no dates, late-night TV? There are no right or wrong answers, only revealing ones. So we'll hold your hand while you take an honest look at your lifestyle, too. Does your job require a lot of business travel? Do you eat out more than four times a week? Are you super social and love to get together with friends for parties, cook-outs, or any excuse to eat, drink, and be merry? Or maybe you're the type that favors dressing down in your most worn-out pair of sweats and throwing open the fridge door, as you pounce on the quickest bites to satisfy your raging hunger? Who are you? What are your food likes and dislikes? What makes you salivate? What makes you gag?

Once you've identified your individual problem times and situations, and can pinpoint what it is that makes you overeat (or do without), they become easier to deal with. And most important, you need to realize that with the freedom to eat more, comes responsibility. Are you ready for that? *The Dish* doesn't mean you can have a splurge-fest on fudge, chocolate chip scones, and croissants. But it does mean you can enjoy all of those foods and other favorites if you just give your meals some forethought (at least as much time as you give to what you're going to wear every day!). It means that you are ready to take full control of yourself and what you eat—eating more of the foods that make you strong, healthy, and full of energy, and less of those that do little but carry an excessive calorie load. By answering the questions in our quiz, you'll know if you have what it takes to succeed at *The Dish*. The key here is self-examination. Have fun with it. Take your time, think before you answer, and be as honest as you can be. (It's just us; come on, whisper it in our ear.) Then check out the Dish Divas' Diagnosis for your answer and find out where to turn to in the book for the Dish on your issues. There, you'll find simple solutions on how you can take control and make a big difference in your diet. Remember, you can be healthy without forfeiting taste or style. This is your first step toward making lifestyle changes tailored to you and your life. The more you know, the more you can eat, and that starts with learning more about *you!*

The Dish Diet Quiz

Time Triggers

Q: **You've just dragged yourself in from a long, hard day. No plans tonight. It's just you and you're all alone with the contents of your refrigerator. What happens next?**

1   You head straight for the kitchen, following the urge to splurge, and man, oh man, everything looks good. You just know how this is going to end.

2   You put on blinders to everything else, and head in the direction of the healthy snacks you've stocked in your kitchen cabinets and begin your routine of weighing and measuring every morsel you intend to put in your mouth.

3   You strip and head for the shower, giving yourself time to unwind and relax, then contemplate over a glass of wine which *amuse bouche* to indulge in before you decide on dinner.

The Dish Divas' Diagnosis

1 If you find yourself scarfing down whatever's on hand in the late afternoon or at night, you're not alone. Even we strong-willed women who make it through the day unscathed can find food cravings in the late-afternoon and evening hours just too much to bear. That wheel of Camembert and leftover baguette that you wouldn't have dreamed of munching on during the day is like a magnet. One slice is too much, but once you get started, ten aren't quite enough. Go ahead and blame it on fatigue, fluctuating hormones, depression, a really, really bad day, or just plain old habit. Whatever the cause, identifying and recognizing when you're most likely to throw caution to the wind and eat whatever tastes good is half the battle. If you know you're eating too much of the wrong foods, but can't quite put a finger on when is your weakest time, keep a food journal, jotting down not just what you eat, but what is driving you to eat. (Journaling can be an eye-opening experience—does your journal reveal you're using food as an emotional rescue? Does it fill a void? And it can zero in on your dietary Achilles' heel—chips, chocolate, muffins, café latte with whipped cream—in short order.) And as much as possible, clear your cabinets of high-sugar, high-fat munching foods (there's no reason to tempt fate) and have a cache of healthy foods at the ready.

2 Okay. You're good. *Too* good. We hate to be the bearer of bad tidings, but there are actually scientific studies that show that people who become obsessive about what they eat, even when it's all good, are actually more at risk for gaining weight farther down the road. All that steel will has to break sometime and it won't be pretty.

3 Now you're talking. Okay, maybe this is an idyllic scene. If you notice, there's no one else, not even a dog, demanding your undivided attention when you walk in the door. But you get the drift. The idea is to do something to shift your focus from food and find your own way to dissolve some of the day's tension before you succumb to temptation. What's that? You say you can't resist the siren call of the fridge? Hey, even Odysseus found a way to resist the hypnotic call of those sexy temptresses. Okay, so he tied himself to the mast, but you don't have to go that far. See what works best for you, and stick with it. Just took a shower this morning? What about perusing the latest issue of a celeb rag? Or listen to that new CD (away from the kitchen).

✳ *Want more?* **Check out chapter 4 for The Dish on Eating In and chapter 8 for The Dish on Cheating.**

It's All Relative

. . . .

Q: Are you cursed with fat genes?

1   Your mom is overweight.

2   Your dad is overweight.

3   You're overweight.

The Dish Divas' Diagnosis

All we care about is if you answered (3). Okay. So your hips are wider than you wish (just like Mom) and you wish you were four inches taller (than your mom). And your dad has a real spare tire. But, hey, you didn't get to pick your parents. You work with the raw materials you've got. We can't all be Jennifer Aniston or Cameron Diaz. You might as well accept your inglorious DNA heritage and take it from there. You can't change your inherited tendency to put on pounds any more than you can change the color of your eyes. But you can work with and around it. (That's why colored contact lenses were invented!) Don't be fatalistic. Your family tendency doesn't have to be your genetic fate. Your smarts, diet, and lifestyle can overcome any passed-on predilection you have to hang on to pounds. Take what you've got and create your own style and be proud of it.

Life's Little Hassles

Q: You've just lost your job, been dumped by the love of your life, your dog failed to notice the difference between his favorite spot outside and the rug. Maybe all three in one day. What do you do?

1   You head for the nearest ice cream place for a double dip of super fudge caramel swirl with nuts and whipped cream. Once you've finished you feel nauseous and guilty.

2   You quietly plot your revenge.

3   You indulge in a massage, you head for a double-feature of those foreign flicks you've been dying to see, you plan a weekend trip to your best friend's for a heavy dose of talk therapy.

The Dish Divas' Diagnosis

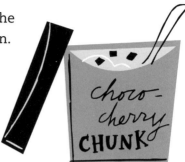

1 Well, you did have a *really bad day*. And splurging like this, while not great, isn't the end of the world. So you fell off the wagon. No big deal. Just pick yourself up, brush off your new snappy, strappy stilettos, and start again. Stop mentally flogging yourself for your ice cream indulgence. A little oral gratification won't hurt (as long as your life isn't a series of life-altering disasters). If you experience a temporary slump because you feel guilty (and nauseous) because you overate, and anxious (and nauseous) over the big, fat consequences, keep telling yourself, "This too shall pass." And it will.

2 Revenge is indeed sweet and best of all, it's calorie-free. But forgive poor Fido. He was having a bad day, just like you.

3 If you have the means and the opportunity for any of the above, go for it. These solutions might sound a little too perfect to be true, but the point is, find what works for you. Consider any and all options that won't add any more to your calorie load.

Is TV Your Trigger?

. . . .

Q: You've planted yourself in front of the tube for an evening of vegetation. (Whatever your secret pleasure, the latest reality TV series, old Joan Crawford flicks, or vintage Japanese sci-fi—to each her own.) What happens next?

1 TV, for you, is fattening. Every time a commercial comes on, you're up and in the kitchen, scrounging for something to eat. The food commercials are the worst.

2 You bring a limited amount of pretzels or popcorn to the sofa and indulge your craving for salty snacks, while you indulge in your craving for trash TV. You're so thirsty by the time the next commercial comes on, you quench your thirst with a cola (you keep a stash on hand for emergencies).

3 When you watch TV, you only watch TV. And when the commercials come on, you find something else to do. When you feel your stomach rumbling, you head for the kitchen and pick from all the healthy stuff you have to choose from.

The Dish Divas' Diagnosis

1 Watching food commercials is like watching gorgeous men and women seducing each other on screen. You can't watch all that smooching and heavy breathing without thinking about, well, you know. Okay, maybe you don't bring the box of cookies to the sofa for some serious munching, but when the ads for KFC come on, you're a goner. And the fridge is just a few steps away. What to do? Hit the mute button and use the few minutes of back-to-back ads to do something else—anything else. Pick up that magazine or book and read a couple of pages, finish making that "to-do" list for tomorrow's dinner, or paint your nails. Better yet, do some sit-ups or jumping jacks. Just get the focus off the tube and on to something nonfood related until your show comes back on.

2 Number one: Toss the sodas or at least switch to the diet version. Better yet, how about keeping lemon-flavored seltzers, bottled water, or peach-flavored iced tea in the fridge? Or make this one of your planned snacks and get in another serving of fruit—a six-ounce glass of nutrient-packed grapefruit juice over ice. (Carolyn Says: Make mine pink!)

Number two: You shouldn't be eating in front of the tube, anyway. That's a basic lesson in Healthy Eating 101! When you're lost in the story, someone could put doggie treats in your bowl and it probably wouldn't slow you down. But at least you got one thing right; you're better off with a bag of popcorn or pretzels than with a quart of Häagen-Dazs and a spoon! If you really must eat, try a handful of nuts (keep them in the kitchen, so you at least have to get up to go get them), or some appealingly sliced up fruits and veggies with a yogurt dip.

3 We're speechless. 'Nuf said. You've got the situation under control (if you're telling the truth, the whole truth, and nothing but).

What's for Dessert?

. . . .

Q: You've just finished a fabulous meal at one of your favorite restaurants in town, but you really, really need something sweet to top the whole thing off. What do you do?

1   You throw caution to the wind and decide to go all the way, ordering the most decadent thing you can find. (Fried *Mars Bar,* anyone?—yes, it's a real menu item at a little eatery on New York's Lower East Side.)

2   You fight the feeling, watching everyone else ordering from the dessert tray. You feel tortured but superior, sipping on your hot water with lemon.

3   You share a luscious passion-fruit tart with a fellow diner, catering to that sweet craving, and walk away feeling satisfied but not stuffed.

The Dish Divas' Diagnosis

1   Could it *be* any worse? Well, yes, but it's still a setback. If you're going to indulge in possibly *the* most decadent dessert on the planet, you could at least split it two, or better yet, three ways, to minimize the damage. The next time, avoid restaurants that offer such "delicacies" as Fried Mars Bars and you've already won half the battle.

2   Self-sacrifice taken to the extreme almost always comes back and bites you in the butt. It's okay once in a while to feel like you're in control and superior, but try not to let your swollen head stretch your halo. It could come crashing down on you. Might be a better idea to at least sample that dessert—the one that's making you salivate like Pavlov's dog.

3 You may have found the best of both worlds—a serving of self-indulgence, seasoned with a dash of self-control. But better make sure that crust isn't drenched in butter or that cream isn't a part of the filling (no wonder it tasted so good). It's best to ask the chef what goes into those dishy desserts, since it's easy to be deceived. And try to order smart—fruit instead of chocolate, sorbet instead of ice cream.

✳ *Want more?* **Check out chapter 5 for The Dish on Eating Out.**

Name That Craving

. . . .

Q: **You're standing in your kitchen looking for something to eat. This is your third round of checking out the contents of your pantry, the freezer, then the fridge. You know you want something, but what? Does that leftover salad sound good? What about an orange? Maybe a few slices of kiwi? What's your next move?**

1 Nothing really "hits the spot," so that container of leftover Chinese takeout will simply have to do. It's better than digging into that box of Godiva chocolates shoved way in the back of the refrigerator. (Out of sight, but not out of mind?)

2 You're not in the mood to cook anything. Even warming leftover kung pao chicken seems like too much of an effort. So, you head for the quart of cookies 'n cream ice cream sitting front and center in the freezer and dig in.

3 Through sheer willpower, you run the Godiva and cookies 'n cream gauntlet and settle on an apple, feeling proud of yourself for making such a healthy choice, even though it does little to diminish your growing craving.

The Dish Divas' Diagnosis

1 You could do worse, but don't make a meal of it. If Chinese food is what you're craving, a few bites should tame the urge without pushing your calorie intake over the edge. If it's not, it could end up just being an appetizer to the real object of your desire.

2 There's just something about a quart of ice cream sitting in the freezer . . . it actually seems to be calling your name! The attraction is like a moth to a flame, as they say, and just as self-destructive. Do yourself a favor and don't keep quart-sized frozen confections on hand. If you must have ice cream at the ready, opt for the individual servings (you know, the kind you were served at birthday parties as a kid, with those impossible-to-eat-with, woody-tasting, so-called spoons) and limit yourself to one. A better alternative is to keep frozen fruit bars on hand for those emergency cravings. Or, go retro and keep a stash of Fudgsicles on hand. (**Densie Says:** Save the banana-flavored for me!) Okay, so they're not quite as rich and creamy as the real thing, but you'd be surprised how suitable a substitute they can be.

3 You made the kitchen rounds. You should know by now if something healthy, like a piece of fruit, is going to work on your craving. If yes, what about tearing into a bag of prewashed Caesar salad greens and go ahead and sprinkle on the croutons and the Parmesan cheese? Now, how about adding other veggies like baby carrots or tasty grape tomatoes? And who knows . . . maybe all the tossing and crunching into those crisp veggies will be positively therapeutic and help you ride the wave of your craving. Yes, croutons, cheese, and salad dressing have calories, but don't forget you're getting fiber and vitamins and you've probably come out ahead calorie-wise compared to taking a dip into the ice cream carton. If all that healthy stuff still doesn't sound good, then you probably weren't hungry at all. Note to self: Learn the difference between hunger and "a cappuccino with biscotti sure would taste good right about now." It's not always easy to know the difference. It's a skill that takes practice. But, hey, you've got time!

✳ *Want more?* **Check out chapter 8 for The Dish on Cheating.**

Good Morning, Mary Sunshine!
· ·

Q: **The sun's not up yet, but you are. The coffee is made (gotta love those automatic timers!) and you're ready to face the day. But first things first—time to break your overnight fast. Not big on breakfast, you say? Don't have the time? What's your morning mode?**

1   You can't face food so early in the morning. Coffee will have to do until your taste buds wake up and your stomach has taken down the "do not disturb" sign.

2   You're an early riser. Always have been. You like watching the sun come up and having some quiet time to read the paper before the activities of the day kick into high gear. Part of that early-riser gig is to eat breakfast.

3   Getting up with the sun is definitely not you. You savor every delicious moment of slumber you can steal. You have just enough time in the morning to grab something before you leave home and scarf it down in the car, bus, taxi, or subway on the way to work.

The Dish Divas' Diagnosis

1 There's no sense forcing yourself to eat early in the A.M., if the body just says no. But if you're up with the sun, you've got plenty of time for your taste buds to warm to the idea of food. If you've been skipping breakfast more often than not, your mother's words should be ringing in your ears: "Breakfast is the most important meal of the day."

Eating in the A.M. recharges your batteries, giving fuel to your brain and your muscles, making it less likely you'll succumb to a mid-morning munchies episode. If you're new to the idea of breakfast, take it slow, but be adventurous. Anything is fair game, if it's healthy. You can try more traditional fare, like scrambled eggs and whole-wheat toast or opt for last night's leftover Greek salad or California rolls, if that's what sounds good. Just try to make breakfast your new good habit. It will make choosing the right foods and not going overboard the rest of the day that much easier.

2 More power to you, if you enjoy getting up early. Now take advantage of your unique body clock and use that extra time to make a nutritious breakfast. (**Densie Says:** My motto—I literally have it hanging in my kitchen—is "All happiness depends on a leisurely breakfast.") Whip up a vegetarian omelet, whole-wheat French toast, or a boiled egg with a toasted English muffin. Top it off with some fresh-squeezed orange juice (all it takes is an inexpensive, plastic juicer and a few oranges). Yum!

3 Since you're obviously not a morning person, and eating on the run is a fact of your busy life, just accept it and work around it. You're not about to whip up a mushroom/onion omelet or even wait for oatmeal to come to a rolling boil. Never fear; quick is okay too, as long as it's something that serves as a nutritional down payment for the rest of the day. Don't reach for sugar-laden breakfast bars or low-fiber breakfast cereals that try to lead you astray with healthy, wholesome-sounding names. Read labels and choose something that provides you with a healthy dose of fiber (at least 3 grams per serving), a minimum of sugar (no more than 3 teaspoons per serving—4 grams sugar = 1 teaspoon) and, if you're not taking a multivitamin, is fortified with vitamins and minerals. As long as you're going the cereal route, be creative and beat cereal boredom by mixing two or three different kinds of cereals in your bowl. (Carolyn loves crunchy Grape-nuts mixed with chewy Raisin Bran. Densie's top breakfast cereal combo: shredded wheat, sprinkled with honey crunch wheat germ.) There are plenty of other good, speedy alternatives. Try instant oatmeal packets that come to life when mixed with a cup of water heated in the microwave. (Tear, zap, pour, and *voilà*, breakfast is served!) Make it with skim milk or soy milk for an extra nutrition punch. Look for whole-grain frozen waffles that you can drop in the toaster, breakfast drinks that provide vitamins, minerals, and fiber along with a third of the calcium you need for the day. And grab a banana, an apple, dried fruit, or grapes to take with you as you dash out the door.

✳ *Want more?* **Check out chapters 4 and 5 for The Dish on Eating In and Eating Out.**

The Dish on Your Diet

Do You Know When to Say "When"?

· ·

Q: You're halfway through your meal. You're not famished anymore, but you're not really full either. Do you know when you've had enough?

1 You know it's time to stop eating when your plate is empty. It's a leftover vestige from dear old Mom and her admonitions to "think of the starving children in China."

2 You make sure that you dish up only half as much for yourself as you would for anyone else. You limit your intake, so you can cut calories.

3 You fill your dinner plate with small servings of meat, large servings of whole-wheat pasta, vegetables, salad, and a whole-grain roll. But you fill up about a third of the way through. You couldn't eat another bite.

The Dish Divas' Diagnosis

1 So you've become a lifetime, card-carrying member of the clean-plate club? It may have served you well when you were a skinny little kid and your mom was concerned you weren't eating enough to fuel your growth spurts. But now you're all grown up and the only way you're going to grow is out. It's time to join the lean plate club and get smaller plates! (Size *does* matter!) It's a behavior modification trick that's been around forever and it really works. If the plate is smaller than your typical dinner plate, you're forced to dish up less and the brain tells the stomach that you've eaten a whole plateful of food. But you wouldn't have to resort to playing mind games with yourself so that you'll eat less if you dish up lots of eat-more foods like brown rice, vegetables, lentils, topped off with a whole-grain roll. If that's what's on the menu, then grab that dinner plate and dish it up!

2 If it works for you and you're not just deluding yourself and following up with second helpings of your micro-servings, then go for it. You should be forearmed, however, with comebacks to comments like, "Is that *all* you're going to eat?" "Are you on a diet? Oh, pleeze! You don't need to lose any weight!" Try: "Me? Diet? No way!" Or you can try the ever popular, "I ate a huge breakfast [or lunch]. Believe me, if this was being served two or three hours from now, I'd be eating twice this much."

3 You are one with our eat-more philosophy. When you fill your plate with all the right stuff, there's little room left for the foods that are slackers in the nutrient department and weigh you down (literally) with an excessive calorie load. And don't forget to take your time eating and drink a tall glass of water (sparkling, bottled, or tap—as long as it's H_2O) before your meal, garnished with a tangy twist of lemon or lime. Bottom line? When you eat more of the right foods, you actually end up with fewer calories.

✳ *Want more?* **Check out chapter 2 for The Dish on Diet Basics.**

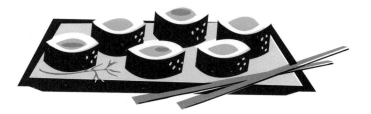

Get Off Your Derriere!

. . . .

Q: How much do you move? A lot, you say? Okay, check it out: Do you take the elevator, even though the door to the stairwell is always open? Do you park as close as you possibly can to the store, the office, the supermarket, even when the weather is great? (Admit it, you'd use valet parking if they had it!) Do you consistently make an effort to minimize effort? Why take two trips (to the car, up the stairs, to the bedroom) when you can do it in one?

1 Oh, yeah. This is you. Why take four steps, when you can take only two? Why get up to get a cup of coffee, when someone just offered to bring it to you? You drop a bath towel on the floor and decide you'll pick it up later. Why in the world would you park at the far end of the parking lot when there are plenty of spaces just a few steps away from the entrance?

2 Well, maybe yes, maybe no. You're no sloth and no one has ever described you as a couch potato, but sometimes you just feel like your get-up-and-go just got up and went.

3 No way. You're always up and movin'. Friends and family marvel at your energy level. You seldom sit and if you do sit, you can't sit still. Fidgeting is just a fact of your life.

The Dish Divas' Diagnosis

1 Whoops! Sounds like you have an undiagnosed allergy to activity. You need to turn your current philosophy on movement on its nasty little head. Think calories, not convenience. A calorie burned is a calorie gone forever; you can kiss that bad boy good-bye! And every calorie-burning movement counts. Take the stairs at the airport instead of the escalator. Waste steps at home. Make

two trips upstairs to get what you need, instead of one. Those seemingly small and insignificant movements can add up. Even bending over to pick up that dropped towel is an opportunity to stretch and tone.

2 Maybe you're no slug, but if your energy level is not exactly at its peak and could stand a boost, you'll benefit from being more active, not less. On those days when you think submitting yourself to a painful flogging would be more enjoyable than going to the gym (at least you wouldn't have to move!), that's your signal that you *need* to go. Not only will it get your blood pumping, studies clearly show it can lift your spirits, making it that much easier for you to face the challenges of the day (dietary and otherwise). Unless you have some undiagnosed health issue that's draining your energy, it's guaranteed you'll feel better, rather than worse, once you've gotten active again.

3 So, you're one of those Nervous Nellies (the ones bobbing their knees up and down under the table). Lucky you. Research shows that you and others like you actually fidget away calories and tend to have an easier time of it when it comes to preventing weight gain. But that doesn't get you off the hook completely. Strength training to keep upper body muscles toned is a must and a little heart-pumping activity should still be on your to-do list, to keep you mentally alert and keep your cardiovascular system in good shape.

✳ *Want more?* **Check out chapter 3 for The Dish on Superfoods and The Dish on Looking Fabulous in chapter 9.**

Holidays: Occasions for Overindulgence?

. . . .

Q: It's _____ (Thanksgiving, Christmas, Hanukkah, Easter, Passover, birthday, anniversary, Mardi Gras, SuperBowl, vacation)—you fill in the blank—and food is everywhere. It's only once a year; what could it hurt to throw caution to the wind and eat all those mouthwatering dishes? What's your approach?

1   Your philosophy is *carpe diem!* You want to grab the gusto, so you grab whatever strikes your fancy on the buffet and savor every delicious mouthful. Where's the joy in living if you can't stimulate your senses and take advantage of every opportunity afforded you? The only way to get rid of temptation, you say, it to give in to it. Self-deprivation is so overrated. (You'll worry about the big fat consequences later.)

2   You make a conscious decision to let loose on some special occasions, like Christmas, and keep your impulse to overeat under control on others, like birthdays. You allow yourself a little decadence, without totally giving in to the dark side.

3   For you, it's all or nothing, so you opt for nothing. Self-restraint is the order of the day, no matter what the occasion. So, you miss out on all those comfort foods. At least you didn't overdo.

The Dish Divas' Diagnosis

1 With that philosophy, there won't be a lot more days left to seize! Food is one of life's joys, to be sure, but you need to get a grip on your *carpe diem* approach to eating. There are ways to deal, without giving in to every twinge of temptation. You need to get your priorities straight and decide which of these holidays are can't-miss in your mind. And if it's vacation that's at issue, remember, excess calories turn to excess pounds whether you're overindulging in Paris or Poughkeepsie. On those holidays you decide you just can't miss, you can let loose and enjoy, as long as you don't replace *all* your eat-more foods with those that positively flash "proceed with caution."

2 You're the solution for the *carpe diem* crowd. Do a good deed and have someone who fits the seize-the-day profile shadow you during the high-temptation holidays and follow your example.

3 Well, well, what have we here? Vying for first place in a self-deprivation contest? First prize: an empty plate? You're either a saint or you've gone over the edge. Resisting temptation is a good thing . . . up to a point. Resisting the urge to eat anything you find especially appealing on special occasions is a setup for feeling sorry for yourself and creating a rebound effect. (On the rebound from the table, where you ate almost nothing, you land with your head in the refrigerator, making a move on the leftovers.)

✳ *Want more?* **Check out chapter 7 for The Dish on Entertaining.**

The Ever-Popular Eyes vs. Stomach Matchup

. . . .

Q: You're eating out—something you do at least four or five times a week. Still, it always feels like a special occasion. You've been so crazed today, you just grabbed a breakfast bar on the way out the door, and barely made time for takeout soup and crackers at your desk . . . and you're starved! What's for dinner?

1 You throw caution to the wind. You deserve a reward today, big time. When the waiter arrives and rattles off the specials of the day, *everything* sounds awesome! You'd take one of each if you could. It's Mexican fare tonight and you start off with a giant frozen margarita, and chips and chile con queso dip as an appetizer. Then you move on to three-on-a-plate chicken-and-cheese enchiladas supreme with sides of refried beans, rice, guacamole, and sour cream and top it off with a delightful little serving of flan for dessert. Hey, some places even have deep fried ice cream for dessert. How about another margarita? It feels so good to be bad!

2 You're into deprivation dining and even the smell of warm tortillas wafting from the kitchen can't melt your steely resolve. You order grilled chicken, with no sauce in sight, pinto beans with no cheese, and unadorned rice. No guacamole. No chips. And certainly no chili con queso. You order ice water with a lime wedge and stare at your friends' margaritas. You leave feeling like you've dodged the bullet.

3 Mexican is one of your faves and one of the hardest to resist. And you know if you don't at least taste some of the good stuff, you're going to feel like you've got an itch you just can't scratch. You order the light version of a Mexican beer and toast your friends! You'll skip the chips. Just too tempting. Or maybe you'll take a

few, put them at your place, and know that's your chip quota. You ask if you can get half portions or a child-size plate of the enchiladas and request a light touch of sour cream. Same good food, just smaller portions. And you skip the flan, since you're already satisfied. Maybe you'll top the meal off with some strong, sweet Mexican coffee instead.

The Dish Divas' Diagnosis

1 With your schedule of eating out, if you throw caution to the wind every time the urge strikes, you've got some serious weight issues ahead. If you've had a stressful day and you know you're going out to eat Mexican, when Mexican food is the weak link in your food chain, then plan ahead. Drink plenty of water during the day and grab something to take the edge off your hunger just before you get there. No healthy foods in sight? Surely, you can find some bottled water? A small bag of peanuts? An individual bag of pretzels? Anything to quiet those hunger pangs and dampen your enthusiasm for ordering everything on the menu.

2 What's the fun in eating out, if every meal feels like a battle of wills (you against your evil twin—the one that wants to indulge and enjoy)? If it feels like an all or nothing battle, and deprivation dining is the only way for you to win the war, then hey, we don't want to change what works for you. But if eating out has morphed from an occasion for celebration into a nightly battlefield, then something's gone wrong. Either seriously consider altering the eating-out aspect of your lifestyle or give yourself a break and enjoy some of what your *café du jour* has to offer. There are ways to enjoy the occasion and still keep your steely will intact. [*check out option (3)*]

3 Atta girl! Compromise, compromise, compromise. Hmmm. Sound like your relationship with your significant other? That's because this is a relationship too! Your relationship with food. And as in any relationship, you can't have your way all the time. Some things you know are good for the relationship (smaller portions of high-fat, high-calorie foods) and others can be destructive (overdoing on chips and splurging on flan, when you're already full). And it never hurts to add a little spice to keep things interesting. (I ask you, what's a Mexican meal without salsa? Salsa, green or red, is a great way to add flavor to any Mexican dish, and give you more taste satisfaction for less.) **Carolyn Says:** I always opt for grilled chicken or beef. Fajitas with green peppers, tomatoes, and onions are a good choice. Then I go easy on the cheese, guacamole, and sour cream, but heavy on the salsa and grilled veggies.

✳ *Want more?* **Check out chapter 5 for The Dish on Eating Out.**

Fast-Food Frenzy

. . . .

Q: Okay, admit it. Even a dish like you resorts to fast food once in a while. This is one of those times. You're on your way home and you know there's nothing in the fridge worth eating. Every day you drive by the best America has to offer in fast food, but today you're going to the drive-thru. The menu board is huge. It's easiest just to order a double cheeseburger and fries, instead of scouring the list for healthier alternatives. It's your turn at the talking box and you're on the spot. What's your plan?

1 A cheeseburger and fries it is. Might as well get the package deal that includes a large drink. (I'll have a number-three combo, please, and could you supersize it?) You're not planning on eating the whole thing, anyway.

2 You never, ever partake of fast food. As far as you're concerned, fast food is fake food. You'd rather spend an extra few minutes making a pit stop at the supermarket to pick up some Italian-seasoned rotisserie chicken (you'll have plenty of chicken left over to make another meal), a bag of prewashed, precut salad greens, and whole-wheat rolls. And you plan to toss some rice with a pinch of rosemary into the rice maker.

3 You're prepared. You bought a nutrition guide to fast food long ago and have already zeroed in on the best. You're not settling for simply the best of the worst, you've actually discovered that some popular fast-food chains have such healthy fare as veggie burgers, grilled chicken salads, and grilled chicken sandwiches (ask for extra lettuce and tomatoes). Hamburgers are a fine choice too, if you don't load them up with bacon, mayo, and cheese. And practice saying these three words, "Small fries please."

The Dish Divas' Diagnosis

1 What is it about a fast-food drive-thru? You always succumb to the smell of French fries. And bear in mind that in the lingo of fast food, "large" often means gargantuan. But there are better choices to be had. Forget about the cars behind you. If you're not sure what the healthier options are, ask. There's a real person on the other end of the squawk box that takes orders all day and is intimately familiar with what they have to offer.

Maybe there's a grilled chicken sandwich you didn't notice, or a green salad without a lot of cheese, or a bean burrito, *sans* the cheese and sour cream. And you don't have to give up your burger and fries; just skinny-size it. Go for the kids' meal with low-fat milk (1 percent or skim if they have it). There's no twelve-and-under rule for ordering kids' meals at fast-food joints. You satisfy that urge to splurge without diving into the fast-food pit.

2 Good for you. This is one time that deprivation is a good thing. Nothing wrong with "depriving" yourself of fast food, especially if you've already got a healthier alternative planned out. But if time is the issue here, maybe you should check out some of the healthier (and quicker) alternatives that some fast-food chains now offer, like baked potatoes (without an overload of toppings), chili (with more beans than meat), spicy grilled chicken sandwiches, veggie burgers, and yogurt. Next time, you can eat healthy and still save time.

3 We're impressed. You already know about those healthful alternatives at some fast-food chains and come prepared to make the best of it. No pressure. You already know the best and the worst on the menu. You've got it under control—nutrition overload averted and with time to spare.

✳ *Want more?* **Check out chapter 5 for The Dish on Eating Out.**

Taking Your Show on the Road

Q: You're traveling this week and it's become a blur of airports, hotels, and taxis. Your usual eating schedule is totally out of whack and you're having a hard time picking the healthiest choices from less-than-appetizing options at airports and the huge serving sizes dished out at the hotels. You're spending so much time getting from here to there that there's no time to plan ahead for healthy meals. What's your traveling diet plan?

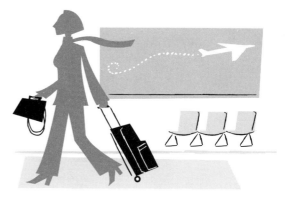

1 No plan. No time for a plan. Your suitcases are bulging, because you threw in everything to cover all fashion contingencies, and you're running late. The taxi is outside honking and you've got to make one last bathroom pit stop before you head for the airport. You know that if you get hungry, there are plenty of restaurants, snack bars, and fast-food franchises to fill you up. You're outta here and on your way!

2 You know the airline food really bites, even if you are "lucky" enough to be on a flight with a meal. And the options at airport food malls aren't much better. Your choices seem to be fast-food burgers, cinnamon rolls, pizza, and jumbo-sized servings of frozen yogurt. You think you're better off waiting until you get to your hotel and have a better chance of ordering something healthy.

3 You're a prepared traveler. You know that even if the airline serves a meal, it's not something that is going to tempt your taste buds or that fits into your healthy lifestyle. And if your flight is food-free, as most are these days, you'll be so starved by the time you touch down that you'll overdo at the first sight of food. So, you've packed snacks and bottled water to help you make it through the next few hours.

The Dish Divas' Diagnosis

1 No plan? Maybe you like to fly by the seat of your pants. But you should be prepared for a crash landing. Flying these days can mean long lines and big delays. That translates into missed meals and forsaken snack times. Not the best scenario for someone trying to eat healthy. You say you had no time to prepare? How long have you known about this trip? Unless you just found out about it two hours ago, there's no excuse for not tossing a few healthy snacks into your carry-on bag, along with some bottled water or 100 percent fruit juice. If you just can't bring yourself to plan ahead, at least be aware that most airport food is high-fat and the servings far too large. And fruits, veggies, and whole grains are rare finds. Think before you order. Stand back from the crowd and check out the options. While there may be slim pickin's in the healthy food department, there are some better options for you to choose. Become familiar with airport food fare and be on the lookout for grilled chicken sandwiches, large green salads, with dressing on the side, crispy tacos with hot sauce, turkey subs with lettuce and tomato. You'll start your trip off right and you'll feel better for it.

2 Get a grip. Maybe holding off until you get to your destination might work in a perfect travel world, where you're always on time. But in today's traveling atmosphere, you're really gambling if you hold off on eating until you get there. You could easily miss a couple of meals and a snack. By the time you get to your hotel room, everything on the room service menu will make your mouth water. And hotels aren't known for their petite serving sizes or their prompt room service—you could end up raiding the snack bar before your food ever arrives.

3 See? That wasn't so hard. Yes, indeed, you're a woman on a well-planned mission. A few well-chosen snacks can make the difference between tolerable travel and the torture of trying to ignore hunger and the headache you feel creeping up on you from lack of food. You've even made room in your suitcase for running shoes and a swimsuit. Who knows? The hotel may have a pool (if you're really prepared, you've called ahead and you already know about the exercise facilities) and you can grab a few wake-up laps before you head to your morning meeting. Your snack stash includes a few small bags of roasted almonds for an energy boost and even some tea bags, so you can use the hotel room coffeemaker to heat up some water and have a relaxing cup of chamomile tea before bedtime, instead of raiding the snacks in the hotel room fridge.

✳ *Want more?* **Check out chapter 5 for The Dish on Eating Out, and chapter 10 for The Dish on What to Eat Today and Every Day.**

What Say You, Dish?

Now that you've taken the quiz, do you see room for improvement? Lots of improvement? No biggie. There's no winning or losing here, no right or wrong. Do you see your food habits in a new light? Was it flattering? Whether your answers reveal you to be the queen of overindulgence, the poster child for self-deprivation, or some combination in between, we think we can still dish out some helpful info that will enthuse, encourage, enlighten, and inspire you to be the dish you know you can be. Even you got-it-under-control eaters can learn a thing or two.

Remember, every day is another chance to eat right when you've chosen to eat healthy for life with *The Dish*. No matter how you answered the questions, we can help. We have the solution and are prepared to share it with you in these pages. We guarantee it'll boost your nutrition IQ, transform you into a confident eater, and maybe even provide a few grins along the way.

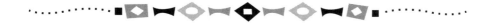

2 The Dish on Diet Basics

You're nobody's fool. You know that staying slim and trim is a direct result of eating less and moving more. But does that mean a life of tofu on toast? Endless lunches of bean sprouts and yogurt? Two hours a day at the gym? Of course not! We want to save you from a life of boring diet plates and self-sacrifice. In this chapter we lay out the basics on nutrition, so you have the food facts to fight back when someone claims fried calamari is the devil in disguise. We tell you what to eat and why—but we promise not to go on too long about the why.

If you're tired of complicated eating plans that ban your favorite foods or order you not to eat certain things after noon (or was that before noon?) and you've tried fasting, but fainted, then start your new food life here with our Dish Diet Basics.

First, we're going to give you a rundown on the nutrition basics that address your unique wants and needs as a real woman with a busy life. Then we're going to get down to specifics. How to be passionate about produce, recognize the healthy carbs, sneak some soy into your diet, get your fish fix, and more. If there's a secret to lifelong weight control and having the energy you need to live your life, then it starts with some smart suggestions for you to adopt and make your own. *But first, let's go back in time.*

This One's for You, Mom

Check it out. After years of nutrition research, looks like Mom was right all along! Hey, even her fashions are back. You didn't think you were the first to wear capris, did you? So, in celebration of moms on a mission to get us to eat right, we present our Retro Rules! Expanding beyond the ever-popular parental plea "Eat your vegetables," they hold just as true today as they did when you were a kid—maybe even more so, now that you're all grown up and having to step up to the plate, so to speak, and take responsibility for your meals.

The Dish Divas' Retro Rules!

1 **Eat your breakfast**—When Mom said breakfast was the most important meal of the day, she was right on target. Turns out eating in the A.M. may slash your risk of weight gain by as much as 50 percent!

2 **Clean your plate**—If you eat a decent meal, chances are you won't be hunting for snacks all afternoon or staring into the refrigerator later on tonight. Of course, the plate is filled with the right foods, right?

3 **Pay attention to what you're eating**—Whether you're watching TV or checking e-mails, mindless munching can lead to overeating. Make the meal the main event.

4 **Don't spoil your appetite**—Stick to some kind of food schedule. If you are hungry way before dinnertime, maybe you should have

eaten lunch. And if you devour a smorgasbord of cheese and crackers before dinner, snacking research shows that you may be full, but chances are you'll still eat your whole dinner out of habit.

5 **Don't wolf it down**—Take time to savor the flavors on your plate. You're dining, not hooking on a feed bag. And the faster you eat, the more you are likely to consume; that's the key to winning a pie-eating contest, not losing weight.

6 **Don't fill up on junk food**—Salty, sweet, crunchy, and full-of-nothing-but-fat-sugar-and-calories junk food sure tastes good going down. But it crowds out nutritious foods and *you'll* end up feeling like junk.

7 **Don't be afraid to try new foods**—Try it, you might like it. Or you might not. It's a taste test, not a commitment. Besides, the more variety in your diet, the more types of nutrients you'll get. And let's face it, variety is a good thing.

8 **Don't eat dessert until you finish your dinner**—Don't fill up on high-fat, sugary foods that lack healthy nutrients before you get your fill of the real thing. Eat your vegetables and whole grains first, then move on to the apple pie.

9 **Learn to share**—The simplest and most effective way to cut dessert calories or any splurge dish by 50 percent is to split it with a friend! Mealtime Math 101.

10 **Go outside and play**—Lying around after a big meal is the worst thing you can do. Even if it means leaving the dishes in the sink, head outside for some fresh air and a walk. Visualize yourself enjoying a stroll down the Avenue des Champs-Élysées after dinner. That's one of the reasons French women stay slim!

Nutrition à la Carte

Why'd Ya Have to Go and Make Things So Complicated?

We debated whether or not to dish out the down-and-dirty nutrition basics. The truth of the matter is, unless you're a real nutrition freak, it can be a snooze-fest. Nutrition science—the real nuts and bolts of nutrition—can have you slipping into dreamland faster than you can say phospholipids. But, we figured no respectable book about healthy eating would be complete without it, so here it is, jazzed up and slimmed down.

All Calories Considered

We're going to cut to the chase on this one: Calories are a simple matter of balance—calories in (from food) have got to equal calories out (what your body uses for energy) or you're left with a flabby surplus (or less likely, a deficit). About two-thirds of those calories are used just to keep your body going—your heart beating, your lungs breathing, and your temperature at a steady 98.6 degrees. What is a calorie? The answer may surprise you. Though you simply may be dying to know how many calories are in that chocolate mousse, the truth is it doesn't actually contain any calories at all. Your body actually produces energy, in the form of calories, from the food you eat. Think of it this way: You need wood and a gas starter to get a fire going in the fireplace, right? Either one by itself is not going to generate heat, but put them together and badda bing, badda boom, you've got yourself a roaring fire. It's the same with food. You've got the chocolate mousse and you've got your body. But you have to put them together to create energy in the form of calories.

Experts quibble over whether some types of fats or carbs are more readily used as energy or, on the flipside, more easily stored as fat. And research suggests that there probably is a difference. But the exact formula for perfect calorie control hasn't been banged out just yet, so our best advice is to digest the basics we've dished up for you, follow our guidelines for healthy eating, keep an eye out for portion distortion, and the calories will take care of themselves.

Count Your Own Calories

. . . .

Here's a universal nutrition truth for you: Everyone's calorie needs are different. While 1,500 calories a day may do you just fine, your best friend may need 2,500 a day to keep her weight on an even keel (that lucky lady!). Whatever calorie charts you might run across in the diet book *du jour,* be sure to take them with a grain of salt. Formulas for figuring calorie needs are flawed, at best, and misleading at their worst. Our approach is less number-obsessed. If you want to lose weight, then you're eating too many calories and burning too few. The next step is a no-brainer: Cut back on food and exercise more. Then, make adjustments if you find you're eating too much or too little. And remember, your calorie needs drop on their own about 2 percent every decade. It may be a drag, but it's a fact of life, so figure 2 percent fewer calories when you're thirty-five, compared to when you were twenty-five and another 2 percent drop when you're forty-five, compared to when you were thirty-five, and so on.

Important calorie info: Don't take too big a calorie plunge. While it's awfully tempting to dive in and go as low as you can for the quickest results, your efforts may backfire, even if you're putting in exercise overtime. Though it may not seem like it at times, your body is a well-oiled machine designed for self-preservation. Once calories drop below a certain level, which is different for everyone, your body kicks into its super fuel efficiency mode and conserves energy at all costs. The result? The number on the scales may not budge, despite a big drop in food intake. Remedy? Add back a few calories (no joke!) but not too much—200 to 500 a day, depending on just how low on calories you've gone, and exercise more.

The 100-Calorie Rule

If you simply must have a number before you can proceed, James O. Hill, Ph.D., from the University of Colorado, Boulder, has one for us— 100. He did some fanciful calculations, based on national surveys of people's weights and calorie intakes, and charted the results. His conclusion? If everyone would get rid of just 100 calories a day, most of our issues with weight gain would be, well, nonissues. "Just cutting 100 calories a day would stop weight gain in 90 percent of the population," says Hill. And, he says, you can split it 50/50. Fifty fewer calories from food and 50 more calories burned with exercise. The best part of all, you're not giving up anything, just cutting back. So, what does it take to cut 100 calories? **Densie Says:** I chatted with my friends and coworkers at *environmentalnutrition.com* (I guess you'd call that my day job) and they agreed to share some of their best tips for cutting 100 calories a day, give or take a few, and we combined them with some of our own.

✳ Enjoy two pieces of whole-grain toast instead of a medium bagel (200 vs. 300 calories).

✳ Portion your pasta. Trim your serving to one cup instead of one-and-a-half cups (280 vs. 420 calories).

✳ Choose a medium baked potato over a large one (160 vs. 278 calories).

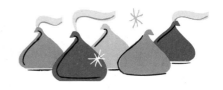

* Eat five Hershey's Kisses instead of one Hershey's Chocolate Almond Bar (128 vs. 230 calories).

* Skip the cheese on your burger (105 calories per slice).

* Top your pasta with a light marinara sauce instead of a cream sauce (120 vs. 240 calories per cup).

* Have two chocolate sorbet bars instead of a mere half-cup of premium chocolate ice cream (160 vs. 270 calories).

* Have a small 4-ounce glass of wine, instead of a larger 8-ounce glass (80 vs. 160 calories).

* Use 1 tablespoon less butter or oil throughout the day (100–120 vs. 200–220 calories).

* Replace one 10-inch flour tortilla with two 6-inch corn tortillas (106 vs. 227 calories).

* Don't supersize your soft drinks. Order a 12-ounce child-size drink over a 21-ounce medium (110 vs. 210 calories).

* Have a 4-ounce T-bone steak, instead of a 5-ounce T-bone steak (365 vs. 455 calories).

* Drink four ounces less soda or bottled, sweetened tea a day (save 100 calories).

* Request skim milk for your two-double-lattes-a-day habit, instead of whole milk (85 vs. 150 calories).

Can We Talk Protein?

Meat, poultry, and seafood, the main sources of protein in your diet, are usually the foods that get star billing on the dinner plate. But these entrées have had their fair share of negative attention too, when it comes to food safety and nutrition. With constant headlines about mad cow disease, the spread of antibiotic resistance, chickens contaminated with bacteria, and mercury in fish, what's a health-conscious girl to do? It's not a one-answer-fits-all kind of solution, but there are some general guidelines we can offer. (For deeper dish on these purveyors of protein, check out chapter 4, The Dish on Eating In.)

For all its popularity, you might be shocked to find out this little-known nutrition nugget: Protein is no higher up in the nutrition pecking order than any other nutrient, despite some spectacular promises made for high-protein diets. Another news flash: It's not

protein per se that you need, but the individual amino acids that link together to create the proteins in foods. (Nine of these are what we nutrition-types call "essential"; you have to get them from food. The rest, the body is able to conjure up on its own.) Oh, one more little-known point about protein: Experts say that protein, not fat, is the nutrient most likely to leave you feeling satisfied after a meal and the least likely to have you scrounging around the kitchen two hours later for something else to eat. A little protein on your plate can go a long way to keeping hunger at bay.

The nutrition powers that be at the Food and Nutrition Board in D.C. have declared that for most women, 46 grams of protein a day is plenty. That's the amount in about one egg for breakfast, 2 ounces of tuna for lunch, and 4 ounces of beef for dinner.

Whether it comes from tofu or prime rib, protein provides 4 calories per gram (112 calories per ounce of pure protein). But don't forget that, in food, protein seldom stands alone. It's almost always mixed with fat (beef, chicken, poultry, and fish) and sometimes fat *and* carbohydrate (most dairy products, dried beans, and soybeans). By the way, most Americans consume 75 grams of protein a day, so chances are slim you'll be lagging behind.

❋ **Please Pass the Tofu** If you've been giving serious thought to making the switch and becoming a vegetarian, that would pretty much take care of all your meat, poultry, and fish issues in one fell swoop. And as any vegetarian worth her sea salt can tell you, meat isn't the only place for protein. Tofu, nuts, beans, eggs, yogurt, milk, and cheese (for almost-vegetarians, who eat eggs and dairy) also rank right up there. Smaller amounts of protein are even found in fruits, veggies, and whole grains. There's no denying that vegetarian diets are healthy—if they're well thought out. (A diet of potato chips and cola is "vegetarian," but certainly not life-sustaining!) The real deal, with lots of fruits, veggies, whole grains, beans, and other plant foods, is packed with Superfoods that can improve your health.

Those Energetic Carbs

Carbs have been promoted as both the answer to your dieting prayers and the root of all dieting evil. Wrong on both counts. Think of carbohydrates as high-octane fuel for your body. You can get by for a short period of time without it (as your body switches to alternative fuel) or with very little, but don't expect to be on top of your game, mentally or physically. Low-carb diets create brain drain and starve your muscles. Carbs are the chief fuel source for your brain and when the fuel tank is always on empty, you won't get maximum performance. That's why marathon runners have that carbo-loading spaghetti dinner tradition the night before the big race. If carb-rich foods like pasta, potatoes, and bread got a bad name for boosting body weight in recent years, it just might have a lot to do with folks who eat too much of the wrong kind of carbohydrates, like the ones found in white flour, sugar, and soft drinks. Surveys that track what we eat say that a lot of us actually eat more than the recommended nine servings of bread, cereal, pasta, and other starchy foods and most of those servings contain white flour.

All carbs, regardless of their source—plant or animal—fall into one of two classes: (1) **Simple Sugars**, which counts among its members sucrose (the white stuff you sweeten coffee and tea with), fructose (the natural sugar in fruit), and lactose (the natural sugar in milk and other dairy foods), plus things like honey, maple syrup, and high-fructose corn syrup—the stuff that sweetens sodas—and (2) **Complex Carbs**, aka starches, found in potatoes, corn, peas, and whole-grain breads and cereals, and made up of sometimes hundreds of simple sugars strung together. When you eat starchy foods, your stomach breaks apart the string of complex carbs, sending them packing back to the simple sugars class. Eventually, all carbs wind up being downgraded to simple sugars. But your best high-carb food choices are also high in fiber, whether they provide simple sugars, as fruit does, or complex carbs, as whole-grain bread does.

Both simple and complex carbs dish out four calories per gram (112 calories per ounce of pure carbohydrates), just like protein. But it's easier to find pure carbs (sugar, honey, hard candy, sodas) than pure protein. So, how much of your diet should come from carbs and, more important, added sugar? High-protein proselytizers aside, the majority of nutritionists believe that high-carb diets are good—anywhere from 45 to 65 percent of your daily calories (though, if you have trouble with fats in your blood—high triglycerides and the like—you'd be

better off sticking with the low end of this rather generous range).

The trick part of this question is about *added* sugars—the sweet stuff that tastes so good in cereals, cakes, cookies, sodas, and ice cream. Extremists say added sugars should make up 0 percent of your diet. Sugar, they preach, provides nothing but calories—no vitamins, no minerals, no phytonutrients—just empty calories. We say, "Phooey!" Sugar is oh so sweet and decadent. A little bit of judiciously doled-out sweets is part of a life well lived. Remember, we're not going for sugar-free here. It's about a small, but oh-so-enjoyable amount in your total diet. If a touch of maple syrup or brown sugar makes those glazed carrots that much more appealing and gets you to eat your vegetables, then go for it. We like the recommendation from a panel of 30 international experts, who recently pronounced that sticking to less

✳ Sugar as Scapegoat

Sugar may have its issues, but making you fat isn't top of the list. Sugar's biggest sin? It keeps bad company, hanging out with those malcontents saturated and trans fats. Can you say, ooey, gooey chocolate-covered glazed doughnuts? Sugar becomes a prime suspect in helping you put on pounds only if you eat lots of the stuff. If sodas, sweetened cereals, chocolate milk, hard candies, fruit drinks, fruit-on-the-bottom yogurt, and sugary cookies make regular appearances in your diet, then sugar may indeed be to blame for your extra padding. Eating a lot of sugary foods may make you hungrier sooner (so you eat more) and it may even slow your body's fat-burning abilities.

Sugar

than 10 percent of calories as added sugars was the best way to go. Need some real numbers to go with that? If you eat 1,800 calories a day, you could allow yourself 180 calories (13 teaspoons) from added sugars. One teaspoon of sugar provides 15 calories.

So, help yourself to a little sugar in your tea or coffee, and the sugar in your after-meal indulgence won't do you in. But make sodas, lemonade, and sweetened teas (which, *BTW*, usually contain as many calories as a soda) occasional indulgences—less than once a week is a good rule of thumb. Otherwise, they offer little more than the opportunity to blow your daily sugar quota in one fell swoop.

Freewheeling Fats

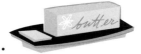

Fat has been the fall guy for everything from weight gain to heart disease, but the real dish on fat is that it's only a problem when you eat too much (calorie overload) or if it's the wrong kind (bad health move). Experts preach everything from low-low fat diets (about 10 percent of calories, where most dietary concoctions taste a bit like tree bark) to higher-fat diets (about 45 percent of calories, a more palate-pleasing proportion). You can find respectable nutrition sorts on both sides of the fat equation. The truth of the matter is, either fat load is probably okay, as long as the fats are of the healthy lot, you're eating lots of high-fiber foods, your sugar intake is minimal, and you keep your calorie intake under control. Ay, and there's the rub! Unlike proteins and carbs, which carry 4 calories per gram, fats pack in 9 calories per gram, making it a double threat if you eat too much. Here are a few fatty examples:

* One tablespoon of oil provides about 120 calories of pure fat.

* One tablespoon of butter or mayonnaise provides about 100 calories of pure fat.

* One tablespoon of heavy cream or cream cheese provides 50 calories of almost all fat.

* One tablespoon of sour cream provides 26 calories of almost all fat.

What's New, What's True

High-fat, low-fat, no-fat?

Can't decide what's the right fat path to take? We only wish it were so easy. There is no right direction. We could just as easily cite the latest research out of Harvard that hints at a higher fat diet being the best for shaving off extra pounds, as we could research out of Europe that shows the opposite—low-fat is best for losing pounds and keeping them gone. So, what's up with that? It probably has a little to do with what turns on your taste buds—fat vs. carbs—and a lot to do with calorie-burning genetics. But since neither the obesity gene nor the gene for fat and sugar cravings has been fingered yet, the best we can offer you is trial and error. If a low-fat, high-carb diet appeals to your senses (you just can't live without, say, penne, potatoes, or pita), try it. But if the taste of olive oil or a sliver of cheesecake is a must, then give a higher fat diet the old college try. One more note: If you're thinking of ferreting out *all* the fat from your diet—get over it. You can't survive on a fat-free diet. Your body demands at least some fat; it's an absolute must-have for every fabulous cell in your body.

Densie Says: My personal preference is a diet with a moderate amount of mostly healthy fat (olive oil, canola oil, and omega-3's). But don't feel the need to count fat grams. It's a colossal waste of time. It's okay if some days turn out to be 45 percent fat and others 20 percent fat. As long as you strike a happy medium overall, you're in good shape . . . pun fully intended.

Fat Family Tree

Our fat-basics presentation wouldn't be complete if we didn't give you the rundown on the fat family tree. Just like proteins are made up of amino acids, fats are made up of fatty acids that can be divvied up into three major groups—monounsaturated (packed in olive and canola oils), polyunsaturated (found in soybean, corn, and safflower oils) and saturated fats (in fatty meats like prime rib and lamb chops and full-fat dairy products like butter, whole milk, whole-milk yogurt, and cream). All types of fat, *we repeat,* all types of fat provide the same nine calories per gram. So while monos may be good for your heart and saturated fats may be bad for your brain, either one can make you pack on pounds, if you eat too much.

✳ **Big Fat Résumés** Not all fats are created equal. They may provide the same caloric punch, but some are better than others for your health. Looking for the right fat for the job? Here's a summary of applicants and what they bring to the table!

Omega-3 Fats—Though actually classified as polyunsaturated fats, generally considered to be in a class by themselves. Work hard at reducing heart disease, cancer, swollen joints, even may help eczema and depression. Found on land and sea in the company of fish, shellfish, flaxseed, walnuts, and canola and liquid soybean oil, has worked in the Mediterranean for centuries keeping generations healthy.

Bottom Line Performance: Lowers bad cholesterol, raises good cholesterol.

Monounsaturated Fats—Long-term experience lowering bad fats and raising good fats in the blood. Also helps manage blood sugar levels. Phytonutrients that travel with monos are an added bonus that may help reduce cancer risk. Monos hold prominent positions in olives, olive oil, canola oil, peanut oil, cashews, almonds, peanuts, and avocados. Most commonly employed in the Mediterranean, where olive oil is the most popular dietary fat. Seeking more opportunities to improve public health worldwide.

Bottom Line Performance: Lowers bad cholesterol, raises good cholesterol.

Polyunsaturated Fats—Although still recognized as a leader in the field for lowering cholesterol levels, demoted several years ago to a less prominent position behind omega-3 fats and monos. Though polys provide healthy fatty acids, including an essential fatty acid we can't live without, they are now suspected of causing health problems if they far outnumber omega-3's and monos. Best when added to the diet in a subordinate position to omega-3's and monos. Chief fat in vegetable oils, including safflower, soybean and corn oils. By far, the most often employed fat in the American diet.

Bottom Line Performance: Lowers bad cholesterol, raises good cholesterol.

Saturated Fats—For decades, held the same low-level position. Known to clog arteries, suspected of underhanded dealings affecting heart health. Chief fat in animal foods—fatty beef, pork, lamb, butter, cream, ice cream, and other full-fat dairy products. Play the heavy, but add lots of flavor to foods; acceptable in small doses. Redeeming quality: Contain a healthy fatty acid called CLA, which is actually sold as a health supplement that may ever-so-slightly help to slow weight gain and boost muscle.

Bottom Line Performance: Raises bad cholesterol.

Hip & Healthy Heroine: Eileen Crane

Fat: Beating the Fear Factor

Carolyn Says: Don't let fat-free and reduced-fat labels rule your shopping list. Rich-tasting foods can add sublime satisfaction to a healthy diet when enjoyed in delicious moderation. "I'm Really Not Afraid of Fat!" That's what Eileen Crane, president and winemaker for Domaine Carneros, told me during my visit to her Napa Valley winery. I wondered how she stayed so fit and energetic while wining and dining for a living. And what a relief to find out that her food philosophy matches ours! She enjoys great meals, and of course great wines, by putting satisfaction first. What's neat about Eileen's background is that she originally trained as a nutritionist and then was bitten by the wine-making bug. So it was off to California to become a winemaker. She joined Domaine Carneros fifteen years ago and now holds the top spot in this beautiful winery, modeled after the grand châteaux of France, looking out upon acres of Chardonnay and Pinot Noir that go into their sparkling wines.

When I first met Eileen Crane, we sipped champagne and sampled caviar, and I wondered, "How does she do it?" (Stay slim and fit, that is.) Because as you can imagine, being in the wine biz requires a whole lot of entertaining. "Socializing is part of my work and it's not unusual for me to have a four-course meal five times a week." Fun yes—but Eileen says when she hit her mid-forties she knew she'd better develop a formula for food and fitness. "I try to walk every day, even when I travel. I walk forty-five to fifty minutes and listen to books on tape." Her food philosophy prioritizes flavor. (Aha! Perhaps that's why she's such a talented winemaker!) "I look for satiety. I don't worry about the hollandaise sauce, especially if it's on really great Napa Valley vegetables." She puts butter on her bread and isn't afraid of the cream in soups. But Eileen is choosy about where she spends her fat calories. She doesn't eat doughnuts or fried foods. And as many of our Hip & Healthy Heroines seem to agree, one square of really good chocolate is so much better than a whole bar of a so-so brand. So, let's raise a glass to Eileen Crane! May I suggest the Domaine Carneros Brut Rosé!

Trans Fats—Ignored for decades, now known to be bad news; long-term experience raising bad fats in blood. Trans position created from the processing of oils into vegetable shortening, stick margarines, and for packaged foods—crackers, cakes, cookies, pastries, cereals. Often travel under the name "partially hydrogenated vegetable oil."

Bottom Line Performance: Raises bad cholesterol.

Tricky, Tricky Trans

Trans fats, those sinister fats that are formed during a process called hydrogenation (code name "partially hydrogenated oil"), and are found in way too many packaged foods, require a minimalist approach. Hydrogenation is as nasty as it sounds. It churns out fats that are as bad, and some say even worse, for your health than saturated fats, which are known to clog arteries to your heart and your brain and maybe even up your risk of some nasty cancers. Oh, and in case you hadn't noticed, trans fats are everywhere. Go ahead, do a quick scan of ingredient labels in your kitchen cabinets for "partially hydrogenated oils." We dare you to come up empty-handed. These funky fats are found in everything from chips, crackers, and cookies to soups, stick margarines, and salad dressings. But we're not advising zero tolerance—it's just too tough to follow a trans-free diet, given your typical supermarket selections, not to mention the fact that foods, even olive oil, contain small amounts of trans fats that occur naturally. But we are giving some hard-core advice (something we usually try to avoid) to read ingredient labels and minimize trans fats in your diet. Your best bet for finding trans-free packaged foods is at your favorite health food supermarket. While regular supermarkets have plenty of trans-free margarine spreads to choose from, you'll be facing one of your biggest dietary challenges yet to dig up choices of trans-free cookies, crackers, and other packaged foods.

Cholesterol—Sidekick associated with bad fats in animal-based foods like butter, cheese, eggs, whole milk, beef, chicken, lamb, liver, and pork. In small amounts, an indispensable part of the body's operation, but known to overwhelm the system and contribute to rising levels of bad cholesterol in the blood.

Human Resources Note: Some people seem to be able to handle cholesterol-containing foods without much of an effect on their blood cholesterol.

Vitamin Vigilance

Quick. What comes to mind when you hear the word "vitamins"? Supplements, right? The "V" word has taken on an almost mystical quality. Take calcium and vitamin D supplements and your bones will last you well into old age; take folic acid supplements and you'll keep your arteries clean as a whistle; take C supplements and cold viruses will bounce right off you. In all the frenzy over supplements—which one is best, how much should you take, how they are regulated—everyone seems to have overlooked one very simple fact: Food should still be your *numero uno* source for vitamins (and minerals—read on). True, if your diet really stinks, you won't come close to getting enough of all the nutrients you need, but if you're making even a halfhearted effort to eat healthy, don't diss your diet . . . it's an indispensable source of vitamins, minerals, and hundreds of other nutrients dubbed phytonutrients. Having laid those cards on the table, you should also know that pathetic diets are way too common—the result of too much fast food, too few fruits and vegetables, not enough whole grains, too much sugar. Which brings us full circle to supplements. They do have a place in *The Dish* philosophy. You'd have to be a die-hard optimist to believe that every day is going to be a perfect nutrition day, so taking a well-proportioned multivitamin/mineral supplement (multi for short) is the perfect insurance policy against a less-than-perfect diet.

Those Phabulous Phytonutrients There's one area where supplements just can't cut it—phytonutrients—those natural disease-fighting, health-promoting compounds found in plant foods. There are thousands, count them, thousands of powerful naturally occurring plant chemicals that give the *raison d'être* for eating all those fruits and veggies. So, if you think you're being smart and taking the shortcut by popping a Vitamin C tablet in the morning to ward off colds and flu instead of drinking your orange juice, think again. You may have outsmarted yourself by choosing the pill over the real thing, 'cause you'll be missing out on all those other healthy compounds orange juice has to offer.

Speaking of healthy compounds—they're secretly stashed away in everything from artichokes to watercress and bear such forgettable names as isothiocyanate and epigallocatechin gallate. But their benefits are important to remember—good health. (For more dish on phytos, check out chapter 3, The Dish on Superfoods.)

Minding Your Minerals

Maybe they haven't gotten the star treatment of vitamins, but minerals are just as valuable to your health and energy. From boron to zinc, they are part of the 24/7 body crew that keeps your bones healthy, your heart strong, helps keep blood sugar on an even keel, and may even help keep you from putting on those extra pounds. Following our sage nutrition advice about what to eat, and putting a daily supplement in your morning routine, will all but guarantee you're getting enough of most minerals.

What's New, What's True
Calcium's Role in Weight Control

The mineral calcium—best known for its bone-building talents—may have a leading role in preventing weight gain. The somewhat radical idea that a mineral could help you manage your weight is all the buzz, even among elite academia types who are generally slow to embrace such unfamiliar notions. Researchers at places such as Purdue University, the University of Colorado, the University of Tennessee, and the University of Hawaii have found that high-calcium chicks tend to weigh less and have lower body fat than low-calcium ladies. They think getting enough calcium in the diet triggers the body to burn more fat and reduces the amount of new fat the body stores. All in all, not a bad deal. And it doesn't take a cabinet-full of calcium to make the difference. In the Hawaii study, an increase of only one serving of a calcium-rich food such as a cup of milk, a thumb-sized piece of cheese, or six ounces of calcium-fortified orange juice—each providing 300 milligrams of calcium—was "associated with" a 2.1 pound lower weight. (That's research-speak for they can't say for sure if the calcium caused the weight difference, but all signs point to yes.) How much calcium is enough? No one knows, though most experts recommend women get 1,000 to 1,500 milligrams a day for overall good health. Best bet? Get your calcium from foods *and* supplements. Just make sure you're getting enough to stack the odds in your favor for stronger bones and a slimmer bod.

Hey, Water Is a Nutrient Too

It's been called the Rodney Dangerfield of nutrients. It's always there, but is seldom given the respect it deserves. After all, you can go without food for weeks, but without the wet stuff, you won't survive for more than a few days. Water ranks right up there with oxygen in terms of body essentials. It keeps your joints lubricated, keeps you mentally sharp (even mild dehydration can drain brain power), helps your body flush out toxins, helps prevent kidney stones, constipation, and urinary tract infections, and even reduces your risk for some types of cancer. Drinking enough water is also important for your skin health—dehydration can make your skin sag and wrinkles look even worse. (Big-time motivation for all you glamour girls!) So drink up for health and beauty! And last, but certainly not least on our list, if you drink it before and after a meal, it just might be able to trick your stomach into thinking you've eaten more than you actually did and put the brakes on going back for seconds.

The most recent potshot delivered against water was from a researcher at Dartmouth Medical School in New Hampshire who decided to trace the roots of the well-accepted recommendation for everyone to drink eight 8-ounce glasses of water a day (8 x 8, as it's affectionately known). It turns out, no one has a clue where it came from, not even the experts. So, should you bail on water? Not a chance. We're big water fans. As a woman, half your body weight is water, but your water level ebbs and flows every day as you breathe, eat, and make regular treks to the loo. If you've got a desk job, go to the gym two to three times a week, you live in a cold weather spot like Minnesota and you're never without a bottle of water in your hand, then you've got the water situation under control. If, however, you're a marathon runner, you spend a lot of even your nonrunning time outdoors, and you live in the Texas heat, for example, then you need even more than 8 x 8, even if you always have a bottle of water strapped to your waist.

Fiber for All

Most fiber comes from plant foods, like beans, broccoli, and oatmeal. It's the part of the plant that your body just can't digest, so it pretty much comes out the way it goes in. There are actually several kinds of fiber, but the two fiber groups you should make a mental note of are soluble and insoluble. Most high-fiber foods contain a mix, but soluble fiber is the main fiber in barley, oatmeal, and fruits like apples, figs, and peaches. Insoluble fiber is the main fiber in whole-grain breads, cereals, and pastas, and vegetables like asparagus, kale, and peas. People who make a living tracking such things say that the average intake of fiber for fabulous females in the good old U.S.A. is a pathetic 12 to 14 grams a day. That falls just a tad short of the recommended intake of 20 to 35 grams of fiber a day. We're not going to pussyfoot around—it's not easy to get that much fiber. But it can be done . . . *if* you know what you're doing. (Check out Dishing Up Fiber on page 55.)

A Tale of Two Fibers

Soluble Fiber: The kind of fiber in oat bran, apples, and beans acts kind of like a sponge in the digestive tract and has been shown to grab onto cholesterol and take it down the line. It's also filling, so it helps keep your appetite in check.

Insoluble Fiber: The kind of fiber in the strings of celery, apple peels, or in wheat bran is indigestible so it works to sweep the intestinal tract clean and keep the "good bacteria" happy. We may run the risk of sounding like a laxative commercial, but we have to say it: Fiber keeps you, ah, regular.

FABULOUS FIBER FIND	GRAMS OF FIBER
Lentils (½ cup)	8
Raspberries (1 cup)	8
Beans, pinto (½ cup)	6
Whole-wheat pasta (1 cup)	6
100% Bran (¾ cup)	5
Dried figs (2)	5
Roasted soy nuts (1 ounce)	5
Almonds (1 ounce)	4
Broccoli (1 cup)	4
Brown rice (1 cup)	4
Dried plums (prunes) (¼ cup)	4
Pears (1 medium)	4
Peas, green (½ cup)	4
Spinach, fresh (1 cup)	4
Banana (1)	3
Oatmeal, instant, plain (1 packet)	3
Strawberries (1 cup)	3
Whole-wheat bread (1 slice)	3
Wild rice (1 cup)	3

Why all the fuss about fiber? High-fiber diets help keep you from suffering crazy highs and lows in blood sugar levels, they help lower cholesterol, prevent constipation, and they may even reduce your risk of some types of cancer. While your body can't digest fiber, the "good" bacteria that are permanent residents in your intestinal tract feast on all that passes by. The result is a bigger, stronger bacterial force that may help keep your immune system healthy. And in keeping with our theme of a happier body, high-fiber diets slow down digestion, making you feel full longer, and delaying the munchies. That makes it a must-have *accoutrement* for every weight-conscious girl's dietary ensemble.

Salt Sense

To salt or not to salt? Whether it's around the rim of a margarita or on top of scrambled eggs, is salt a bad thing to love? If only there was a clear-cut answer. It's the sodium in salt (aka: sodium chloride) that has the image problems. And yes there are enough studies on the health effects of sodium (particularly blood pressure) to fill a salt mine!

It turns out there are experts on both sides of the salt shaker. Some say only those who are "sensitive" to sodium need be dedicated salt watchers. It's a genetic thing. But last time we checked, they weren't offering DNA tests for sodium sensitivity at the doc's office. Still, some very large, impressive studies do clearly show that slashing sodium intake lowers blood pressure in lots of people, but you'd have to go way low on the sodium scale to see any real health benefit. On the other hand, sodium is an important player in the body's fluid balance; too much salt in your diet can contribute to water retention and bloating. Hold the salt on my margarita, please!

To help provide kind of a one-size-fits-all sodium recommendation, experts have issued a blanket rule to limit sodium intake to 2,400 milligrams a day—the amount in 1 teaspoon of salt (salt is only about 60 percent sodium).

Obviously, the more you shake on the salt, the more sodium ends up on the plate. But the real sodium load comes from processed foods like soup and frozen dinners. Just check out the Nutrition Facts panel of the label to see the sodium content lurking inside.

Bottom line for salt lovers? If everything is in working order (no high blood pressure, healthy kidneys, strong heart), we see no reason to be overly cautious about sodium. Just remember flavor comes from the natural goodness of food too!

Densie Says: If you can believe it, I grew up putting salt on watermelon, apples, cantaloupe, even oranges—gag me now! But I eventually learned to enjoy their natural sweetness, without the salt shaker in hand. Moral of my salt shaker story: Even the most salt-dependent taste buds can be retrained to enjoy flavors *au naturel*.

Did Someone Say She Was on a Diet?

Favorite diet quotes of all time.

Densie Says: "O! that this too too solid flesh would melt, thaw and resolve itself into a dew." Okay, so it's Shakespeare, not Nutrition 101, and it falls under the category of wishful thinking, not diet advice. (Any excuse to use that quote.) Still, Will nicely sums up our deepest desires about losing weight. We all wish we could close our eyes, click our heels together three times, and make the extra pounds go away. But since that ain't gonna happen, we've got plenty of easy-to-digest diet advice in the following pages. It's not the eat-a-half-a-cup-of-cottage-cheese-and-call-me-in-the-morning-type advice. We're more of an "antidiet" frame of mind. We truly believe that the more you know about what your food possibilities really are, the more you can eat and achieve eating satisfaction.

Carolyn Says: "I never worry about diets, the only carrots I'm interested in are the number you get in a diamond."—Mae West. Hey we all need a little motivation to make changes in life. And successful dieters who lose the weight they want and keep it off share one common quality—they are motivated. It could be a big reunion or wedding in your future or finally getting fed up and saying good-bye to bad food habits of the past that gets things started. But continued success means making a change on the inside by putting your health first. You are worth it! Take the time you need to go on that walk. Buy those great-tasting right-off-the-vine, organically grown tomatoes for your salad. Reward yourself with a pretty pedicure. You'll glow and it will show. Personal motivation is powerful and research studies show again and again if you want it, you'll make it happen. Hey, keep the diamond on that wish list too!

What about Those High-Protein Diets?

. . . .

But before we get into our dishy guidelines, a word about one of the most popular diet choices these days. High-protein diets have enjoyed way more than their fifteen minutes of fame over the past thirty years, and recent research (funded by the high-protein prince, the late Dr. Robert Atkins) found that high-protein diet devotees were actually able to reduce their cholesterol levels. That said, we still believe high-protein diets, which are by default high-fat and low-carb, are not the best way to go for most people. Despite their long-lived popularity, high-protein diets won't make you forever svelte, healthy, or pump up your energy. To be fair, some of the most popular high-protein diets will help you quickly knock off extra pounds. In fact, high-protein diets are often used in medically supervised weight control programs for the obese to jump-start weight loss. And just ask some of the recent "success" stories. Their enthusiasm is positively contagious. What high-protein diets *aren't* destined to do is help you *keep* off those extra pounds. Go back and quiz those so-called success stories six months or a year after the fact, and see if they're still so enthusiastic about the high-protein way. Chances are, they badly missed the occasional indulgence in a sub sandwich, popcorn, the taste of real sugar in their coffee, honey in their tea, and the impromptu "How about some ice cream?" and returned to the same old eating routine. I mean, how willing are you to *permanently* ration pasta and bread? True, for some people, these diets do work long-term (especially if you're a sirloin and salad kinda gal). But check the fine print on side effects; high-protein diets can cause constipation, bad breath, and irritability—not exactly three of the most attractive qualities a girl would want! So for most, it's not a way to live your life . . . for the rest of your life.

The Dish Divas' Eat-More Rules!

Now that we've served up our Retro Rules on *how* to eat and topped them off with the basics, we're going to dish up our guidelines on *what* to eat for adding more color, more texture, more nutrients and phytonutrients, more variety, more flavor, and more satisfaction to your life. Turns out that good nutrition doesn't mean avoiding a long list of offending foods; it means adding great-tasting health-boosting foods to your day!

They're all here, in the *The Dish Divas' Eat-More Rules*. Each rule spells out why it is so important for your health and provides shopping tips and label-reading guidelines. The overriding theme: The more you cozy up to nature (unprocessed foods), the greater the rewards—count 'em—good health, high energy, a sharp mind, and a happy body.

1 Ya gotta get whole grains! It's not news to a smart girl like you that whole grains are awesome sources of fiber and antioxidants (in the same class as fruits and vegetables). That's important, especially when you consider new research out of California that suggests women may actually need more antioxidants than men. And a whole slew of studies have found that eating a lot of whole grains is good for your health—lowering your risk for heart disease, diabetes, and cancer, just to name a few diseases we would all like to dodge. Think whole grains and you probably conjure up whole-wheat bread, barley, oats, and brown rice, but there is so much more than that. Don't disregard more adventurous whole grains like amaranth, quinoa, spelt, or triticale. (BTW: When you've got the munchies, popcorn and baked tortilla chips are also considered whole grains.) Sorry, but that palate-pleasing polenta you had last night doesn't count. Wild rice, which isn't

Densie Says: Really want to expand your whole-grain horizons? Are you a do-it-yourself kinda gal? Try stone-ground versions of black bean flour, ten-grain flour, fava bean flour, garbanzo bean flour, or millet flour to make breads, biscuits, pancakes, and scones. A great source of old-fashioned, slowly stone-ground flours is Bob's Red Mill: *www.bobsredmill.com*. They do it the old-fashioned way, grinding grains slowly, but surely, between millstones imported from France and Denmark. Not quite sure what to do with those stone-ground ingredients? The website offers hundreds of recipes to get you started on the healthy whole-grain path.

actually a grain at all, but a type of grass, is high fiber, so go ahead and lump it in with whole grains. And that's just the beginning. Why all this obsessing over whole grains? It's about the *fiber!*

The number-one way to jumpstart your fiber intake every day? Dish up a whole-grain cereal for breakfast—shredded wheat, bran flakes, flax flakes, raisin brain—the higher the fiber count of the breakfast cereal (they can range from less than 1 gram per serving, in cereals like puffed rice or cornflakes, to 3 grams in a packet of oatmeal, all the way to 14 grams per serving in an all-bran cereal), the better off you'll be. Top it off with fresh fruit, like sliced bananas or fresh whole blueberries—more fiber topped with more flavor—and you're really on your way to your 20 to 35 grams-a-day goal.

2 Be passionate about produce. Think decadently sweet, juicy melons; just-picked peaches that still smell of the tree; round, plump blueberries the deepest blue you've ever seen. Are you drooling yet? That's the point. If you go for good-quality, fresh produce can be just as enticing as other less dish-worthy choices and, it goes without saying, are loads better for you.

Think of all those vibrant fruits and vegetables as the must-haves in your diet. The more color variety in your choices, the bigger the variety of health-promoting phytonutrients on your plate. Be a fruit and vegetable detective. Move beyond apples, bananas, and oranges. (We're not knocking the big three in the fruit world, but variety keeps it interesting.) Expand your produce repertoire. Enjoy golden kiwi, star fruit, blood oranges, pluots, and loquats. And, in the veggie domain, a gal can't live on green beans and carrots alone. Try out kohlrabi, purslane, watercress, Swiss chard, jicama, and yellow beets. If you try something for the first time at a restaurant and like it, jot down the name and make a beeline to your local farmers' market, health food store, or culinary shop and ask if they can get it and, while you're at it, check out their produce for new varieties. Sophisticated tastes and svelte waists demand variety. Variety in taste, variety in color, and variety in nutrition.

Carolyn Says: I remember visiting the Napa Farmer's Market for a CNN story on why Americans don't eat enough produce and being amazed at the number of different kinds of melons. I was traveling in a newly discovered taste orbit that extended way beyond cantaloupe and honeydew. The farmers offered samples of melons I had never even heard of before. Each melon's flavor burst in my mouth, working its own magic on my taste buds. I envisioned fruit salads composed of nothing but melons—deep orange, pale green, bright green, pale yellow, bright yellow. It became clear to me that the reason most Americans don't eat enough produce is that they're just not tasting the *right* produce!

A Picture-Perfect Pound of Produce

How much is enough? A researcher acquaintance of ours, Dr. David Heber of the University of California, recommends a pound of produce a day. Sounds like a nice round number to us. (It's not as much as it sounds, honest!) Just how much is a pound of produce? You can mix and match to your heart's desire, but each pound of prevention is a good place to start.

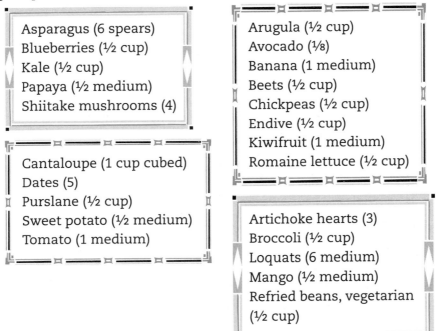

Asparagus (6 spears)
Blueberries (½ cup)
Kale (½ cup)
Papaya (½ medium)
Shiitake mushrooms (4)

Arugula (½ cup)
Avocado (⅛)
Banana (1 medium)
Beets (½ cup)
Chickpeas (½ cup)
Endive (½ cup)
Kiwifruit (1 medium)
Romaine lettuce (½ cup)

Cantaloupe (1 cup cubed)
Dates (5)
Purslane (½ cup)
Sweet potato (½ medium)
Tomato (1 medium)

Artichoke hearts (3)
Broccoli (½ cup)
Loquats (6 medium)
Mango (½ medium)
Refried beans, vegetarian
(½ cup)

✳ Daily Produce Scoop

A tisket, a tasket, here's another way of looking at your produce basket: Aim for five to nine servings of fruits and vegetables a day. A pound or five to nine servings, either way will get you there.

What's New, What's True

Take a Walk on the Raw Side

Densie Says: Raw food diets are all the rage. Ya gotta admit, it's an appealing idea. Such beauties as supermodel Carol Alt and actresses Demi Moore and Alicia Silverstone reportedly like it raw. But should you boycott *your* stove? Enthusiasts (and they are incredibly enthusiastic) say if you eat only raw fruits, vegetables, nuts, and seeds, you'll improve your health, delay aging, and clear your mind. Okay, so here's the dish: Raw foods are great . . . if they're handled properly (bad bacteria could be lurking in raw foods and won't be killed off with cooking) and if you happen to enjoy all your food served at either room temperature or chilled. (Think cold raw vegetables, cold raw main dishes, cold soups and eggless, sugarless, flourless cakes, and, well, you get the picture.) Because eating raw meat is an incredibly bad idea, raw food diets are vegetarian by default. That can be a good thing. But there is no logical reason to believe that raw foods are somehow naturally better for you than cooked. You might be interested to know that research clearly shows that several foods are actually more nutritious when they're cooked. You get significantly more phytonutrients from say, carrots and tomatoes, if they're cooked, compared to if you eat them raw. Our advice: Have a little of both, some cooked, some raw, and splurge on a meal at a raw food restaurant whenever you like. It's fun! Just don't turn yourself inside out trying to adhere to a difficult and unproven raw foods diet.

What's New, What's True

Breaking the Color Code

Densie Says: What's the code? Red, blue, green, purple, orange, and yellow—the eye-stopping colors of fresh fruits and vegetables. The color code decoded? Eat lots of brightly colored fruits and vegetables. Okay, so there is no real secret code to be broken, but a friend of mine, Daniel Nadeau, M.D., an assistant professor at Tufts University, and a practicing endocrinologist, felt that the color of food was so incredibly important for eating well that he teamed up with James Joseph, Ph.D., a heavyweight in nutrition research, also at Tufts, and wrote a book on the subject, *The Color Code: A Revolutionary Eating Plan for Optimum Health* (Hyperion, 2002). Dan says their color code is both simple and revolutionary: Brightly colored fruits and vegetables produce tons of natural plant compounds, called phytonutrients, to protect themselves from the outdoor elements and from disease. When you eat all these plant foods, you're getting a healthy dose of that same protection. The deeper the reds, blues, greens, and oranges of the food you eat, the greater the protection factor. (For more dish on phytonutrients, see chapter 3, The Dish on Superfoods.) And he wanted to make sure to drive home this fact: Only whole foods offer the unique combos of phytonutrients natural to plants. Supplements just can't duplicate that recipe.

3 Get your fish fix. At least twice a week, make way for food that comes from water. Whether it's whole roasted talapia, grilled turbot, fillet of sole with capers, baked flounder, superfresh cod, teriyaki salmon, sea scallops with chili paste, smoked trout, sea bass cooked in white wine (take a pass on Chilean sea bass—it's on the road to extinction), lobster or shrimp gumbo, your body will say thank you. Seafood is your best source for those "healthy" fats you hear so much about, called omega-3's. These special fats have been found to do amazing things for your heart and your mental health. It may even keep your skin looking smoother longer, but there's less evidence to back up that claim. But as long as you're making the effort to reel in some fish on your plate twice a week for your health, you'll have all omega-3 bases covered.

If you've never thought of yourself as a fish lover, then maybe you should try acquiring a taste for it. Sample different varieties of seafood, different recipes and different spices. Fish that tastes fishy either isn't fresh or wasn't prepared properly. (See chapter 4, The Dish on Eating In, for some tips on getting the freshest catch of the day.) But there's a downside to dining from the deep blue sea. Some fish contain levels of mercury that if consumed too often can add up to toxic levels in your body and cause a host of disturbing and dangerous symptoms, from hair loss and headaches to depression and memory loss. Fish found to be highest in mercury content are amberjack, Chilean sea bass, grouper, halibut, shark, swordfish, and fresh tuna. Lowest in mercury content include catfish, clams, orange roughy, oysters, salmon, sardines, shrimp, and tilapia. Flounder, mahimahi, red snapper, and trout rate in the middle.

But, if it isn't open for discussion: If salmon, flounder, tuna, and shrimp will never pass your lips, you might want to consider one of the following also-rans to reach your omega-3 goal.

Another source of omega-3's is alpha-linolenic acid, a fatty acid found in canola, soy, walnuts, purslane, and flaxseed oils. To a certain extent, your body can convert it to the omega-3's you find in fish. But it's a clunker of a system—not a very efficient process and you can't know how much of the omega 3's you're getting out of the deal.

The third omega source is the so-called designer eggs, such as Eggland's Best and Gold Circle Farms, which come from hens fed fish oil, algae, or flaxseed. The hens then dutifully lay eggs that contain one type of omega-3 in greater-than-normal amounts, but nowhere near as much as you get from fish or supplements.

4 *Take time out for tea.* Surely you've heard the health claims for green tea. "Drink it and you will be healed." At least that's the impression we get from our own nonscientific survey of the coverage. Sounds promising. But what if you've just never quite been able to acquire a taste for green tea? (You're not alone.) The good news is you can feel free to stick with the Lipton or Tetley black tea you've got in the cabinet. Tons of research is now showing that while the types of beneficial compounds found in green and black teas differ, they each may provide health benefits that range from strengthening bones to aiding weight loss (so far that's been studied only with green tea).

Tea experts from around the globe believe that the drink's health benefits may come from naturally occurring compounds called flavonoids. In your body, these antioxidant flavonoids work to mop up harmful molecules called free radicals that, over time, can make you sick. Or, so the theory goes. No one has actually taken people, fed them tea over a period of years, and kept a running log of their illnesses. It would just be too time-consuming and expensive. But lots of research shows that, in general, tea drinkers are healthier than non-tea drinkers. And a recent study hints that tea may also provide a healthy dose of immune-boosting compounds. What's the effective "dose"? Studies have hinted that anywhere from one to ten cups a day may be needed to provide benefits ranging from cancer prevention and cholesterol lowering to strengthening bones, protecting skin, and boosting weight loss. But any amount of tea is probably a good thing, since the antioxidant powers in tea can comfortably go one-on-one with fruits and vegetables. If you like your tea with milk and sugar, don't forget to make a mental note of the calories. While tea is calorie-

✳ Funky, Fabulous Food Facts

The Real Thing

Real tea comes from a specific plant, *Camellia sinensis*. It's more of a bush, really. Herbal teas come from, well, herbs. That puts herbal teas in a whole other category. While they may offer their own unique benefits, depending on the herb, don't lump them in with real teas.

free, the milk and sugar, as we all know, are not. If you're watching your caffeine intake, black tea is like a half-caff cup of coffee; green tea has even less caffeine. Another tea tip: decaffeinating tea may get rid of the caffeine, but it also tosses out much of the flavonoid stash.

5 **You need more nuts in your life.** Despite the high-fat reputation these nutrition nuggets carry, they can also provide some pretty awesome benefits. While nuts are fatty foods (about 12 to 14 grams of fat per ounce), most of that is healthy fat, including omega-3's in walnuts, similar to what you find in fish, and monounsaturated fats like those in olive and canola oils. Whether you choose almonds, walnuts, peanuts, pecans, or pistachios, nuts are rich in protein, fiber, and lots of other nutrients (even vitamin E and calcium!), putting nuts on our nutrition "A" list.

Research shows that people who regularly eat nuts—about one and a half ounces a day, five days a week—are at much lower risk of having their arteries clog than non-nut eaters. BTW: An ounce and a half is a handful, not a canful! Nuts can also help keep your blood sugar on an even keel, and the most attention-grabbing news for calorie counters is that research also suggests that eating nuts may dampen your appetite, putting the brakes on your tendency to overindulge. To add flavor and a dash of satisfaction to salads or cooked veggies, toss in a handful of roasted nuts.

NUTS	NUMBER OF NUTS PER OUNCE
Almonds	20–24
Brazil nuts	6–8
Cashews	16–18
Chestnuts	3
Hazelnuts	18–20
Macadamia	10–12
Peanuts	28
Pecans	18–20
Pine nuts	150–157
Pistachios	45–47
Walnuts	8–11

✳ Funky, Fabulous Food Facts

Goobers Get Down

Peanuts win the Miss Popularity contest hands down (they're the number-one snack choice, when you feel like a nut), but did you know that they're not really nuts at all, but legumes? While they seem to have been adopted into the nut family, they actually share the same genetic pool as beans and lentils. But they're the only legume that gets down—way down—growing underground. Still, for all that nonconformity, peanuts hold all the health promise of any other nut—lower cholesterol, less heart disease, reduced risk of diabetes and best of all, researchers at Purdue University believe that the peanut and its offspring, peanut butter, have the ability to stave off hunger and prevent weight gain.

Here's our "best-of" dish on nuts:

Best antioxidant source: **Brazil nuts**—the single best food source of the antioxidant mineral selenium.

Best omega-3 source: **Walnuts**—rich in a fatty acid that your body converts to omega-3's.

Best fiber count: **Almonds**—about 4 grams per ounce.

Best source of folic acid (B vitamin good for your heart and your overall health): **Peanuts**—provide two to five times more folic acid than other nuts.

Best source of vitamin E: **Almonds**—provide about four to ten times the vitamin E of other nuts.

Best serving size: **Pistachios**—forty-seven nuts go a long way to satisfying your craving for a salty snack.

Best appetite suppressant: **Peanuts**—while the findings for peanuts probably hold for all nuts, peanuts have been studied the most for appetite control.

Best calorie count: **Chestnuts**—only 69 calories per ounce. Most nuts clock in at about 160 to 200 calories per ounce.

6 Sneak in some soy. Okay, we'll be the first to say it out loud. The taste of soy is no joy. But things are improving. (**Densie Says:** However, I'm a convert and snack regularly on roasted soy nuts.) If you've decided to take in some soy, don't get in a tofu rut; think soy milk, soy cheese, soy-based soups, soy burgers, soy dogs, soy sausage, and edamame (those green soy pods served at sushi places), just to name a few. Give them all a try and find one or two that tickle your taste buds.

So, what's so great about soy? The simple soybean is packed with powerful phytonutrients, the most famous being isoflavones, thought to be a real boon to good health. They're rumored to fend off all kinds of diseases like heart disease, osteoporosis, and cancer, and for women "of a certain age," to help relieve the symptoms of menopause. But some say it's possible to get too much of this good thing. Does soy have a dark side? Possibly. The much ballyhooed isoflavones in soy do what they do because they tend to copycat the natural female hormone, estrogen, in your body, but with less impact than the real thing. While a little estrogen is a very good thing for women, too much is a bad thing. The question is, "Can you get too much soy?" If so, "How much is too much?" Researchers are still trying to answer these questions. Our advice is to include soy as one of the 1,000+ pieces to your dietary puzzle. (That's not to say you should be spending hours trying to put the pieces together.) But don't go overboard drinking only soy milk, eating only soy cheese and soy-based meat substitutes, and snacking only on soy nuts and edamame. A little here, a little there— a couple of servings a day is fine—and you'll get the pluses of soy, without risking getting too much of a good thing. For the total lowdown on soy and soy products, check out the Soy Foods Guide at *www.unitedsoybean.org.*

✳ Soy Sauce Shakedown

Despite its name, soy sauce is actually isoflavone-free. So is soybean oil. All those healthy phytonutrients are lost during processing.

Like Beans, Soy Is a Musical Fruit

Soy may seem like a hip and healthy food, but one not-so-cool fact about soy that is seldom spoken—it can give you gas. Not so surprising, when you consider it's a close relative of the bean. Soy, like other beans and legumes, contains undigestible carbohydrates, called oligosaccharides. While you may not be able to digest them, the friendly bacteria that live in your intestinal tract chow down, producing gas as a by-product. Just something to bear in mind the next time you're contemplating whether to order a soy burger at a dinner with friends.

7 **It's all about the oil.** A little oil in the sauté pan or drizzled over salad greens can make or break the dish, but too much poured on can make or break your diet. All oil, we repeat, all oil, whether it's canola, olive, soy, peanut, sesame, or avocado, provides the same number of calories per tablespoon—about 120. (Unbelievable as it may be, butter actually provides a little less—about 100 calories—because it also contains water.) Oil is a good thing for your heart and provides fatty acids needed for overall good health. And it tastes good—pasta tossed with a teaspoon of olive oil, vegetables stir-fried with a swirl of sesame oil. Hey, even if you've got the balsamic vinegar, you can't make a great vinaigrette dressing without the extra-virgin olive oil. So, to maximize flavor and minimize the total fat, be sure to use good-quality oils and discover the high-impact, flavor-infused oils, like olive oil with basil, chile pepper, garlic, cardamom, or a more subtle vanilla (it does wonders for pasta). You can make your own "cold-infusions," as chefs call them. Put some olive oil, peanut oil, or whatever suits your fancy into a blender with shallots, garlic, basil, chives, or freshly grated nutmeg. Hit the blend button and there you have it. Your own oil infused with the flavor of your choice. (See chapter 4, The Dish on Eating In, for olive oil cooking tips.)

8 Be a Spicy Girl! Let loose and experiment with herbs and spices. Flavors are the fashion statements in recipes and when good food tastes great, chances are you'll eat what's good for you! A favorite Middle Eastern saying of ours, "Give to the pot, and the pot gives to you." Translation: Don't be shy with herbs and spices. They provide much more than flavor. As plant foods, they are fabulous sources of antioxidant phytonutrients. Think, but don't limit yourself to, bay leaves, black peppercorns, oregano, thyme, and rosemary. Expand your spice rack to include cardamom pods, fenugreek seed, saffron, turmeric, and whole coriander. They're your culinary ticket to take your dishes around the world, from French tarragon to Indian curries.

Besides herbs and spices being good sources of nutrients, like vitamin C (parsley, cilantro, and basil) and carotenes (turmeric, marjoram, and paprika), the National Cancer Institute has identified celery, ginger, and garlic as containing strong anticancer properties. Mint, rosemary, thyme, oregano, and sage contain antioxidant compounds that may also be a boon to good health. And don't forget that commonly used cooking herbs like garlic and ginger have well-documented health benefits, such as lowering cholesterol and managing gastrointestinal upset. Herb rule number one—Buy fresh whenever you can. Or grow your own in window pots. Want to earn a green thumb? Herbs sprout like weeds. It's a cinch, and just think how suave you'll look snipping fresh basil for the tomato and mozzarella salad you're serving to guests! Order of herbal preference from greatest to least: (1) freshly picked herbs; (2) fresh packaged herbs; (3) dried herbs.

So, take full advantage of your new appreciation of herbs and spices. Once you've gotten the hang of this spice thing, you'll never go back. Check out our chapter 4, The Dish on Eating In, for some herb and spice combinations that can help you whip up some surprisingly tasty vittles without breaking a sweat!

※ **Densie Says:** My two favorite fresh herbs to nurture at home are mint and rosemary. Hot tea with freshly picked mint is simply the best (especially if you're under the weather) and fresh rosemary snapped from the twig (and a little garlic) adds a last-minute gourmet kick to potentially blah foods like chicken and potatoes.

9 H_2O to the Rescue. Research shows that getting plenty of water can help keep your metabolism revved. So, as we said earlier, forget the new water naysayers who are challenging the eight glasses a day rule. Get it whenever you can. Drinking lots of fluids, especially water, is necessary for preventing dehydration in the summertime heat, and studies have also shown that people who drink the most fluids have a reduced risk of kidney stones, bladder cancer, and even colon cancer. One study found that men who drank about ten cups of fluid a day were only half as likely to develop bladder cancer as those who drank less than five cups a day. (We can only assume that the same holds true for us females.) Water drinkers may also have a lower risk of heart disease. The message is clear: Get as much fluid as you can and make the most of good old H_2O. Don't wait until your tongue is sticking to the roof of your mouth, or you'll never make your quota. If you exercise outdoors in the heat, carry a water bottle around with you and take a swig whenever you can.

Water tips: A glass of H_2O needn't be your only water source. Lots of foods, especially fruits and vegetables, add a healthy portion of water to your daily intake.

Food	Percent Water
Fruits/Vegetables	80%–95%
Cooked Cereal	85%
Eggs	75%–80%
Pasta	65%
Fish/Seafood	60%–85%
Meats	45%–65%
Cheese	35%
Bread	35%–40%

. . . And if you're a caffeinated coffee, cola, or tea drinker, the latest from the powers that be at the National Academy of Sciences is that these drinks count too.

(For the lowdown on fancy fortified and flavored waters, check out chapter 6, The Dish on Drinks.)

10 Have a backup plan ... please. Taking a multivitamin/mineral supplement is your insurance policy for those hectic days when you just can't quite seem to eat everything you should. The real simple advice is to look for a name brand multivitamin/mineral (aka "multi") that provides you with 100 percent of the Daily Value (DV) for most vitamins and minerals. It's an imperfect system, but it works pretty well. But don't make selecting the best multi a major project. Trying to pit one brand against another is your classic case of comparing apples and oranges. One brand has more chromium, but less vitamin C; another has more calcium, but less magnesium. Just look for one that seems to provide the most nutrients, without stepping over the line (thumbs down to supplements that offer 500 to 1,000 percent or more of any nutrient). Don't forget that you're still eating a healthy diet that's packed with its own supply of vitamins and minerals. And if you eat a fortified breakfast cereal, you're getting another mini-dose of nutrients, though some, like Total cereals, pack in 100 percent and sort of steal the thunder from supplements, providing as many vitamins and minerals as you'd get in a one-a-day-type pill.

Dish Nutrition Note

Wow! I wonder how many calories you burned just reading this chapter alone! Congratulations! You have just graduated from Dish Nutrition 101. Now on to the advanced application of this newfound knowledge—cooking at home, eating out, even entertaining. You'll see how these food facts form the foundation for our philosophy, "The more you know, the more you can eat!"

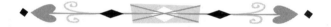

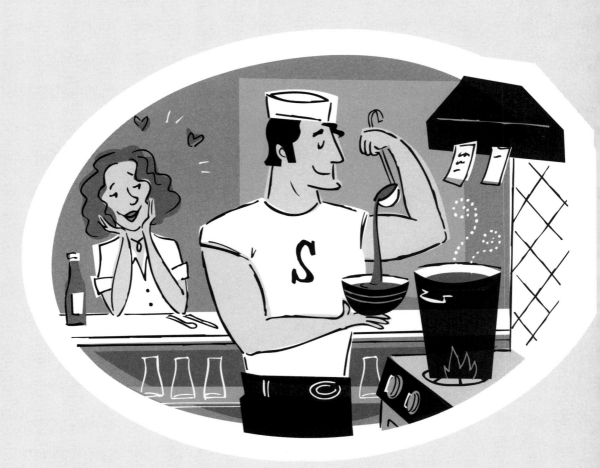

3 The Dish on Superfoods

Just about everything you eat, from a stem of broccoli to a bonbon, contains nutrients that your body uses to keep on ticking. But there are foods in a select crowd that deserve to be elevated into the "Super" stratosphere because they pack a superior punch of vitamins, minerals, and other needed nutrients. These are the foods that nutrition researchers get excited about for their "food-as-medicine" capabilities to treat or prevent what ails ya, from kidney stones to cancer. Dietitians who design weight-control plans love these Superfoods too, because

> An old-fashioned vegetable soup, without any enhancement, is a more powerful anti-carcinogen than any known medicine.
> —James Duke, M.D.

they dish up the most nutrition per calorie. More good news: This list of powerhouse packages from good old Mother Nature includes foods you're probably already eating, like blueberries, orange juice, spinach, and almonds. So read on and eat up!

To streamline things a bit we have chosen some of the top contenders in elite eating and we're going to tell you why they're oh-so-good for you. To qualify for Superfood status they have to be impressively high in one particular nutrient or contain an awesome variety of nutrients—the nutritional equivalent of one-stop shopping!

Phabulous Phytonutrients

Plant foods, including fruits, vegetables, whole grains, beans, peas, and lentils, are packed with phytonutrients—the real secret behind their Superfood status. While they may not be able to leap tall buildings in a single bound, many are believed to help slow aging. Also known as phytochemicals ("phyto" actually comes from the Greek word for plant), these naturally occurring compounds also pack a powerful disease-preventing punch. Superfoods, indeed!

If the names of some of these phytonutrients sound like something you dealt with in Chemistry 101, then check out our "Phabulous Phyto-Guide" for cut-to-the-chase info on what each can do for you. There are hundreds of phytonutrients found in foods. That's why variety is a good thing. The bigger the variety of what you put on your plate, the more phytonutrients you're likely to take in. Oh—and it's worth noting that while Superfoods rate high on health, most just happen to be conveniently low in calories. What more could a girl want?

Phabulous Phyto-Guide

. . . .

Alpha-carotene—the body converts it to vitamin A, though not as much as beta-carotene. Acts as an antioxidant and may help boost the immune system.

Anthocyanins—may prevent urinary tract infections, keep eyes healthy, prevent cancer, help short-term memory.

Beta-carotene—the body converts it to vitamin A; may help prevent cancer.

Beta-sitosterol—proven to lower cholesterol.

Ellagic acid—one of the cancer-prevention gang found in plant foods.

Ferulic acid—an anticancer compound found in whole grains.

Glutathione—sometimes called the "mother of all antioxidants," it's an antioxidant protein that functions in the body as a detoxifying agent, a defender against certain cancers and viruses, as well as an immune cell booster.

Hesperidin—laboratory studies clearly show that hesperidin inhibits the growth of cancer cells.

Limonenes—studies suggest these compounds may have stronger anticancer powers than some anticancer drugs. May also help lower "bad" cholesterol levels in the blood.

Lutein—important for keeping eyesight healthy.

Lycopene—potent antioxidant that may help prevent heart disease as well as prostate cancer and breast cancer.

Phenols—a large group of antioxidant compounds that includes anthocyanins, catechins, rutin, and quercetin.

Quercetin—linked to a lower risk of cancer.

Resveratrol—best known for its link to a reduced risk of heart disease.

Rutin—acts as an antioxidant and may have anticancer properties.

Salicylates—shown to reduce the risk of heart disease. Makes sense, since it's the same compound found in aspirin.

Superfoods: Tall Tales and Fanciful Food Facts

Apples—Eve tempted Adam with an apple, Snow White fell under the spell of a poisoned apple, and each year thousands are lured to the Big Apple to seek fame and fortune. What does all that have to do with apples being a healthy food? Not a darn thing. It just makes apples seem a bit more enticing. They were, after all, the first forbidden fruit. Though the natural good-for-you compounds vary among apple varieties—a Granny Smith will have slightly different phytonutrients than say, a Golden Delicious—apples are generally rich sources of quercetin, potassium, and soluble fiber. And a recent study out of Rio de Janeiro (a place where they should know a thing or two about being slim—it is, after all, the birthplace of the thong) found that eating three apples a day helped women lose weight. Now, you can cross two things off your list (eat more fruit and lose weight!).

1 medium apple = 80 calories

Apricots—cultivated by the Chinese, starting some four thousand years ago, it was believed that the apricot had special fertility-enhancing properties. Today, fresh, dried, or canned, these little golden-blushed nuggets of good nutrition are packed with beta-carotene, vitamin C, potassium, fiber, and antioxidant-powered flavonoid phytonutrients.

4 fresh, dried, or canned in juice = 64 calories

Asparagus—this "food of kings," so knighted because King Louis XIV of France was wild about it, has been touted as a way to ward off bee stings, treat heart ailments, and relieve the pain of toothaches. Asparagus is also said to provoke lust. A seventeenth-century herbalist once wrote that asparagus "stirreth up bodily lust in man or woman," and

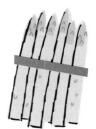

prescribed that it be boiled in wine and eaten in the morning. Whatever turneth you on! It's likely that its purported lusty reputation was due more to its appearance (think about it) than the natural compounds it contains. Now, we just know it's good for you. It's a rich source of vitamin C, thiamin, vitamin B_6, fiber, selenium, and one of the best foods around for the B vitamin folacin. Plus, asparagus has the phytonutrients glutathione and rutin.

7 medium spears = 26 calories

Avocados—the Aztecs believed avocados were an aphrodisiac and dubbed it *ahuacatl* (meaning testicle), a not-so-subtle reference to the fruit's shape and the way it hangs from the tree. Whatever . . . Among the twenty top fruits, it ranks highest in lutein, vitamin E, glutathione, beta-sitosterol, folacin, fiber, and magnesium. All that and a creamy satisfying texture that adds a rich taste to sandwiches and salads.

⅕ California avocado = 55 calories

Blueberries—a former favorite of Native Americans, these midnight-blue berries have since been found to be one of the top fruits when it comes to disease-fighting antioxidants. Talk about a thrill on Blueberry Hill! They contain fiber, vitamin C, and potassium, but the natural phytonutrients found within are what really make blueberries shine. If you can believe it, there's even a research center at Rutgers University devoted totally to researching the benefits of the blueberry, along with its ruby-red cousin, the cranberry. Among big blue's other benefits—it's on the list of foods that help prevent cancer and urinary tract infections, it's being researched for its power to protect short-term memory as you age, and may even help your baby blues (or greens or browns!). In fact, in Japan, blueberries have been dubbed the "vision fruit." The key to all this healthy stuff is a group of phytonutrients known as anthocyanins.

½ cup = 40 calories

Broccoli—this Italian import brought good health along for the boat ride. Broccoli is a member of the brassica family with cousins including cabbage, broccoli rabe, brussels sprouts, and cauliflower. It's being studied for its ability to turn off cancer-causing enzymes in the body, thanks to the phytonutrient sulforaphane. It's also a good source of vitamin C, beta-carotene, potassium, the B vitamin folate, and calcium.

3 spears = 108 calories

Cantaloupe—what we call cantaloupe is actually a muskmelon, and it dates back to biblical times. Even Moses and his gang had a craving for melons, as they trekked across the desert. Wherever you are and whatever you call them, cantaloupes are packed with beta-carotene (the bright orange color is the giveaway) and are good sources of vitamin C and potassium as well.

⅛ medium = 24 calories

Carrots—doctors in the Middle Ages prescribed carrots as a medicine for every imaginable affliction, from syphilis to dog bites. It's no miracle cure, but carrots offer the mother lode of beta-carotene. Beta-carotene, used by the body to make Vitamin A, is important for healthy vision. That's why your mom may have told you that eating carrots was good for your eyes. Cooking makes the beta-carotene even more available for you to absorb. But you can overdo it. If you eat too many carrots (or any food high in carotene) you'll find the palms of your hands and the soles of your feet turning a strange shade of orange. It will look like you used a bad fake tanning cream. No harm done. Just cut back on your carrot intake. Carrots are also good sources of potassium, good for keeping your blood pressure in check.

½ cup = 26 calories

Cherries—European folklore has it that if you repeat this rhyme in an eenee-meenie-minie-mo fashion, when counting the number of cherry stones you have after eating a bowl of cherries, you will know if and when you are going to get married: *This year, Next year, Sometime, Never.* And, of course, the cherry has been long associated with a woman's virginity. We're not sure how that one got started, but we can, with all confidence, say that there is no scientific connection between the two. Cherries are, however, a good source of vitamin C and fiber. The biggest potential health bonanza comes from phytonutrients quercetin, anthocyanins, ellagic acid, and beta-sitosterol, a cholesterol-lowering compound. Cherries are also a top source of melatonin, a compound that the body manufactures and uses to control your normal sleep patterns.

1 cup = 90 calories

Corn—it's the focus of some pretty intense Native American folklore about the beginning of time and such, but for us it's just a great source of the phytochemicals lutein, zeaxanthin, and ferulic acid, with a dose of potassium and fiber thrown in for good measure. Summer sweet fresh corn on the cob is a treat and you really don't need to slather on the butter. Canned or frozen corn niblets add nutrients and fiber to soups.

1 medium ear = 77 calories

Dried Plums (aka prunes)—they're the fruit "formerly known as" prunes. Image consultants, no doubt, wanted to play down prunes' reputation for battling constipation and play up the culinary connection. Dried plums add great texture and flavor to so many foods from salads to baked goods. (Yes, they'll still help move things along when your bowels get a bit sluggish, but so do lots of other high-fiber foods.)

They are also an absolutely amazing source of a group of health-promoting antioxidants, called phenols. In fact, the USDA has ranked prunes number one in antioxidant power. They're also good sources of fiber, potassium, and both alpha- and beta-carotene and a heart-healthy compound known as salicylate—the stuff that makes an aspirin a day *de rigueur* for heart health.

5 dried plums = 100 calories

Fish—yes, once again, Mom may have been right. Fish may indeed be brain food. Studies point to the possibility that fish may help keep your brain sharp as the years go by. Other research just keeps piling up to prove the disease-preventing powers of fish. It's the fat in fish that packs the healthy punch. Together, two omega-3 fats, known in shorthand as EPA and DHA, can help protect your heart (and don't kid yourself—your risk rivals that of a man once you hit your mid-forties). Best fish sources of healthy fats? Anchovies, halibut, herring, mackerel, salmon, sardines, trout, and tuna. (Check mercury concerns info in chapter 4, The Dish on Eating In.)

3 ounces = 110–190 calories (mackerel packs the most calories; anchovies and halibut the fewest)

Flaxseed—ancient East Indian scriptures reportedly said that in order to reach the highest state of contentment and joy, a yogi must eat flax daily. Even Gandhi said that where flaxseed goes, good health follows. Can't argue with those credentials. What exactly are flaxseeds? They are simply the seeds from the flax plant and flaxseed oil is the oil squeezed from the seeds. And it's super in more than one way! Flax is also the plant that gives us linen for that cool, crisp look on a hot summer day.

Flax is one of the richest plant sources of omega-3's (the healthy fat in fish) and lignans, estrogenlike plant compounds that may help fend off breast cancer and help control your blood sugar. If that's not enough, it packs fiber and antioxidants. Grind the seeds up in a coffee bean grinder (or buy premilled flaxseed in a box at the health food store) and toss into casseroles, burgers, pancake and muffin batters, and cereals. And today you can even buy certified organic pastas made with flaxseed that provide a hefty dose of omega-3 fats in each serving.

1 tablespoon ground flaxseed = 36 calories

Grapefruit—whether sliced in half, sectioned in a salad, or squeezed into a refreshing glass of juice, grapefruit offers much more than just the vitamin C that citrus is famous for. It's a good source of potassium and fiber—one half a grapefruit provides six grams of fiber. (No, you don't have to eat the peel!) And studies have shown that grapefruit can help you cut calories by curbing your appetite. The chewable fiber in the pulp, plus pectin, a softer fruit fiber, has been shown to contribute to satiety—that full feeling you get after a meal. So grapefruit is a good food to eat when you want to be trim. Ruby red grapefruit offers even more nutrition—the pink tinge indicates the juice contains beta-carotene and a host of other colorful nutrients.

8 ounces juice = 100 calories; ½ grapefruit = 38 calories

Kiwifruit—a study out of Rutgers University declared this New Zealand native (though much of it now comes from sunny California) to be the most nutritious fruit around; it's packed with vitamin C, lutein (for healthy eyes), fiber, potassium, and copper. A ton of nutrition in a rather homely fuzzy brown package. Slice it open though, and you reveal the green glory of the slightly tart kiwi. Golden kiwi, which still hails from New Zealand, offers similar nutrition and is sweeter than green kiwifruit.

1 medium kiwifruit = 46 calories

Mango—this seductively sweet and aromatic fruit from the mango tree is considered a symbol of love in India and some believe the mango tree can grant wishes. Maybe, but we promise it *will* grant you super nutrition. As you savor this succulent fruit (which is actually *the* most widely consumed fruit in the world!), remember that it's packed with beta-carotene, vitamin C, potassium, and fiber. And make a couple of wishes, while you're at it.

1 medium mango = 135 calories

Down on the Farm

Just because most of our Superfoods are from the vegetable kingdom doesn't mean there aren't some super things to say about meat and dairy. Bear in mind you can get too much unwanted cholesterol and saturated fats in the mix, but there's also some super stuff inside. Lean red meats, such as beef tenderloin, serve up healthy amounts of vitamin B_{12}, iron, magnesium, zinc, just to name a few of the major players. Milk (and we're talking skim or 1 percent, to avoid the bad stuff) is a great source of calcium, phosphorous, and vitamin D, needed for strong bones and pretty pearly whites. (And don't forget calcium's possible role in making weight loss just a tad easier.)

Eggs are another much maligned animal food. But it just so happens that eggs are the gold standard when it comes to protein. In fact, egg protein is so complete and digestible nutrition scientists consider it the "reference protein" against which all other proteins are measured. Eggs are also a respectable source of iron, vitamin A, vitamin D, and the B vitamin riboflavin, and even the phytonutrient lutein, found in the yolk. Downside: 213 milligrams of cholesterol per egg, contained in the yolk—if you're counting such things. That's why egg-white omelets are a healthy choice. Add some chopped spinach and mushrooms and you've created a "super" dish.

Nuts—almonds, hazelnuts, pecans, pistachios, walnuts, and peanuts. If you've blacklisted any of them because you thought they were fattening, they're all worth reconsidering. Packed with vitamins, minerals, and phytonutrients, they are calories well spent. And the oil inside is the heart-healthy kind. Walnuts are particularly good sources of omega-3's; almonds are a good source of protein, calcium, magnesium, and vitamin E; Brazil nuts contain near-supplement levels of the mineral selenium (strongly believed to fight cancer) and some nuts boast hearty amounts of resveratrol, a phytonutrient found in wine that may be behind part of its health benefits. And the research suggesting nuts are good for your heart is strong enough to support a health claim approved by the FDA that "eating one and a half ounces per day of most nuts as part of a diet low in saturated fat and cholesterol may reduce the risk of heart disease." (That's about a third of a cup, or a handful.) And nuts such as almonds, pecans, and walnuts have been shown to actually help you control your weight because they can curb your appetite between meals. (See chapter 2, The Dish on Diet Basics.) So grab a handful (not a can full) and be a real health nut!

1 ounce nuts = 160–200 calories

Orange Juice—whether you squeeze it yourself or buy it by the carton, orange juice is the number-one Superfood beverage. It's positively packed with vitamin C, a great source of vitamin B_6 and B_1 and potassium, and it sneaks in a shot of magnesium as well. Not to mention its stash of several healthy phytonutrients such as limonenes and flavonoids. The phytonutrient hesperidin, found within, may be a major player in the fight against cancer.

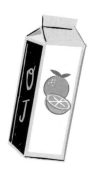

8 ounce glass = 110 calories; 1 orange = 65 calories

Raspberries—it's been said that raspberries were originally white. That all changed, according to legend, when the nymph Ida pricked her finger as she picked berries for her infant, Jupiter. Ever since that day, raspberries have been red with her blood. So much for legend. But the fiber content of raspberries is itself legendary, with a whopping 8 grams per cup (more than a lot of so-called high-fiber cereals). Yes, the fiber is in the seeds! They're also a good source of vitamin C and vitamin B_6. On the phytonutrient front, they can strut their stuff about ellagic acid and anthocyanins, both of which are powerful antioxidants.

1 cup = 60 calories

Soy—as far as we can tell, the soybean originated in China and took its own sweet time (a couple of thousand years) to make the trek to the United States. And now it's here to stay. But whether you're talking about tofu, miso, soy burgers, or edamame, you either love it or you hate it. For soy lovers, soy is the richest source of isoflavones you can put on your plate. These phytonutrients are renowned for their health-promoting properties and pack a powerful antioxidant punch. Diets rich in soy may help manage your blood sugar and cholesterol levels, reduce your risk of several kinds of cancer, and for women, help with the symptoms of menopause. Two or three servings a day is good, but more than that and you're entering uncharted territory. The very compounds that make soy a healthy food could actually pose health risks if you go over the edge with your newfound soy enthusiasm. (For more about soy, see chapter 2, The Dish on Diet Basics.)

1 tablespoon miso = 35 calories
1 cup soy milk = 81 calories
½ cup edamame = 100 calories
¼ cup roasted soybeans = 136 calories
3 ounces tempeh = 197 calories

Spinach—all worn-out references to Popeye aside, spinach was a Superfood before nutrition was considered cocktail conversation. It's a native of Iran, but today Alma, Arkansas, population 3,000, has been dubbed "The Spinach Capital of the World" (based on what, we're not exactly sure), complete with an annual Spinach Festival. Not only is spinach rich in beta-carotene, fiber, magnesium, vitamin K, and the B vitamin folate, it contains other phytonutrients that may slow brain aging. And there was actually a study that found spinach eaters were more likely to preserve eye health.

½ cup cooked spinach = 21 calories

Strawberries—rumor has it that Madame Tallien, a prominent figure at the court of the Emperor Napoleon, bathed in the juice of fresh strawberries. It took twenty-two pounds of berries to fill a tub. Needless to say, she did not bathe daily. The ancient Romans believed that strawberries alleviated symptoms of melancholy, fainting, inflammation, fever, throat infections, kidney stones, bad breath, attacks of gout, and diseases of the blood, liver, and spleen. Now, we neither bathe in it nor believe it is a cure-all. But strawberries are an excellent source of vitamin C, the B vitamin folate, potassium, fiber as well as flavonoids, anthocyanidins and ellagic acid. Strawberry fields forever!

1 cup strawberries = 50 calories

Tea—we've already sung the praises of tea in these pages, but a list of Superfoods simply wouldn't be complete without it. Drinking tea has been linked to a reduced risk of stroke, heart disease, and some types of cancer. It may lower cholesterol and boost the immune system. And green tea may rev up your metabolism, helping you burn off a few extra calories a day, if you drink enough of the stuff. All these pluses are probably due to the high levels of phytonutrients known as catechins found in all teas—black, green, oolong, and white. Add a squeeze of lemon, sweeten with dark honey, and you've got a phytonutrient gold mine in every cup. And a little known fact about tea is that it also offers you a bit of vitamin K (only recently tagged as an essential vitamin for strong bones) and magnesium, which has a long-standing reputation as a bone-builder.

1 cup brewed tea = less than 5 calories

Tomatoes—the French have referred to it as "The Apple of Love," the Germans "The Apple of Paradise," but the British believed it was poisonous and avoided it completely. That fear was carried over with the early settlers and we didn't begin to appreciate the tomato until the early 1800s. This juicy, sweet summertime fruit (yes, it's a fruit, not a vegetable) is one of the top sources of the newly appreciated phytonutrient lycopene, which is being researched, as we speak, for its potential to reduce the risk of heart disease, prostate cancer in men, and breast cancer in women. It's another good source of vitamin C and potassium. Like beta-carotene, lycopene is actually more available in cooked foods than raw. So, don't dismiss tomato sauce, tomato juice, tomato paste, salsa, or even ketchup (though it has a whole salt-and-sugar thing going on) as excellent sources of this powerful phytonutrient!

1 medium tomato = 25 calories

Whole Grains—not so long ago, unprocessed brown bread was considered something for peasants who couldn't afford the more pure and pristine white breads. Talk about your flip-flops. Now, it's the brown breads that are pricier. But they're worth the cost. Whether you're talking about whole-grain cereals, whole-grain breads, whole-grain crackers, or whole-grain pasta, they all have one thing in common: They are made with 100 percent whole grains and are packed with lots of the good stuff that will bring you good health—magnesium, fiber, vitamin E, selenium, lignans, ferulic acid, flavonoids, phytates, saponins. Eating whole grains has a clear connection with less heart disease, diabetes, and cancer. Now you have another reason to "eat the whole thing"!

1 slice whole-grain bread = 80–100 calories
½ cup whole-grain pasta = 98 calories
5 whole-grain crackers = 85 calories
¾ cup all-bran flakes = 92 calories

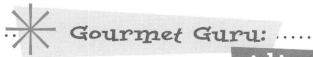

Gourmet Guru: Alice Waters

Truly Superfoods

Back in 1971 when Chez Panisse restaurant opened in Berkeley, California, very few people knew about organically grown foods or had even heard of heirloom tomatoes, free-range chickens, or fava beans. But Chez Panisse served it all up in a four-course menu that changed every night. In a city where social change was the tune of the time, Chef Alice Waters started her own revolution—a revolution in taste and health. Still going strong today, Chez Panisse continues to win culinary accolades from fans who crave the earth's best, served with elegance.

We asked Alice for her definition of Superfoods. She quickly responded that superior quality is what makes foods super. Great-tasting tomatoes or peas or corn are a result of choosing varieties bred for their culinary characteristics and then planting them in the best soil, tending them carefully, and, Alice adds, "harvesting them at the peak of ripeness so you can bring them to the table with an aliveness. I don't want foods that have been in a plastic bag for a week!" Alice, known for her alchemist skills in the kitchen, and for her ability to capture even the most delicate flavors in food, says surprisingly, "How it's cooked, comes last."

Carolyn Says: I remember visiting Alice Waters on the twenty-fifth anniversary of Chez Panisse for a profile on CNN and found her outside the kitchen all excited because a delivery of vegetables had just arrived. "They're from Chino Farms near San Diego. I never know what they'll send because it depends what they've picked this morning." You would have thought they were all boxes from Tiffany's! She leaped about, prying them open to reveal the treasures inside—darling tiny green beans, bouquets of multicolored radishes, glorious heads of curly endive. And then the mushroom forager walked up the drive. She called to greet him and couldn't wait to see what he had found today. Oh, there would be morels on the menu tonight!

So, to find true Superfoods you have to be superdemanding about where you shop and what you buy. And voting with your fork, Alice believes, is the best way to promote the highest-quality foods with supertaste and supernutrition. That just happens to be super for the earth and the small family farm. *Suggested reading: Chez Panisse Vegetables* (HarperCollins, 1996).

Hey, We're Super too!

Mother Nature may have started it, but more than a few smart humans have cooked up ways, with a little modern ingenuity, to improve the nutrition profiles of certain foods, catapulting them into the supercategory too. Foods like orange juice with added calcium, cereals fortified with lots of vitamins and minerals, and yogurt with good-for-you active bacterial cultures are all souped-up versions of their former selves.

Not So Super

While many of these Superfood creations are great additions to your healthy diet, some of these "man-made miracles" are a waste of time and taste. Marketers looking to pull a fast one and make a quick buck try to borrow the "health halo" of a truly good food to make the new version of the original look better in a shopper's eyes. They're kind of like guys who look cute at first, but then ooze with bad pickup lines. Don't be fooled: Oat bran beer is not a healthier choice, and Saint-John's-wort may be an herb linked to better moods, but Saint-John's-wort–laced potato chips won't get you there. The deal is that there's usually nowhere near enough of the good ingredient in the product to give you the health advantage you're looking for. Bye, guys!

A Sampling of Man-Made Superfoods

Cereals—Whole-grain cereals can stand on their own healthy merits, but most cereals today are fortified with a supplement-like list of vitamins and minerals. Some even include omega-3 fats, flaxseed, and soy sprinkled in for good measure. Just remember that if you choose a cereal that provides 100 percent of the recommended daily intake of a nutrient, you're basically getting a supplement in cereal form. Taking a supplement pill that provides another 100 percent is just doubling your intake. True, there aren't many cereals that go that far with the added vitamins and minerals. In fact, most typically provide about 25 percent of the recommended daily intake. *FYI*: At the other end of the spectrum are cereals you might see at your local health food supermarket. While many are whole grain and some come from soy, spelt, flax, and oats, making them healthy choices, few brands have the levels of vitamins and minerals added that you'll find from major brands in the supermarket. Is that good or bad? Depends. If you're already taking a multivitamin/mineral supplement, then you really don't need more vitamins and minerals from your cereal. If, on the other hand, you've limited your food intake and you count on every food being jam-packed with nutrients, then maybe a highly fortified breakfast cereal is just what the dish diva ordered.

Fortified juice—**Densie Says:** Before calcium-fortified juices hit the market, if someone had asked me what I would think about fortifying orange juice with calcium, I would have cocked my head to one side, raised one eyebrow, and exclaimed incredulously, "Do what?" But it turns out it was a stroke of genius. What a nifty way to get more calcium in your diet, especially if you're not a milk drinker. How much calcium are we talking about? You get a glass of milk's worth of calcium (about 300 milligrams) in every eight-ounce glass of juice. Some even now boast extra vitamin C, added vitamin E and vitamin D. You can't beat that!

Teas—in its natural state, tea qualifies for Superfood status. But while it's a great natural food, it's also been morphed into a man-made Superfood. You can find bottled teas fortified with a wide range of amino acids, herbs, and nutrients that promise to do everything from calm your nerves to help shave off extra pounds. Our take on these tanked-up teas? Don't mess with Mother Nature! (For more on tea check out chapter 2, The Dish on Diet Basics, and chapter 6, The Dish on Drinks.)

Energy and Supplement Bars—Think! bars, PowerBars, Tiger's Milk Bars, Balance bars, Met-Rx bars, Boost bars, Prozone bars, Soy Sensations bars. You name it, you got it. There's a bar for every function: high protein, high energy, brain power, muscle building, weight loss. Are they food supplements worth seeking? If they're taking the place of something like a chocolate candy bar, then, yes, they do offer a nutrition edge of added vitamins and minerals and, sometimes, fiber. But they also tend to offer lots of sugar, calories, and even saturated fat. Some, like Luna bars, billed as "the whole nutrition bar for women," are lower in calories than most because they're— smaller (1.7 ounces, though it's still a good choice)! So, if you read labels carefully and choose wisely, they can be great for grab 'n go meals. Just don't make it a regular thing.

Raising *the* Bar

There are a few bars that rise above the rest, because they are low in added sugar and saturated fat and offer up a decent dose of fiber (at least 3 grams). Here are a few suggestions. The calorie counts will vary a bit, depending on the flavor.

Boulder Bar	200
Clif Bar	240
Luna Bar	180
Odwalla Bar!	250
PowerBar	250
Soy Sensations	180

Yogurt—To carry the "yogurt" name, a product has to contain a certain number of so-called "good bacteria." These bacterial good guys, which actually sound scary, include *L. casei*, *L. bulgaricus*, *L. reuteri*, and *L.*

acidophilus, some of which normally reside in your intestinal tract. However, providing reinforcements, in the form of probiotics (foods or supplements that provide live, active bacterial cultures) can help do everything from fend off a common nasty side effect of antibiotics (diarrhea), defend against infections (maybe even nasty yeast infections), and possibly boost your body's defenses against more serious diseases, such as cancer. Yogurt is also a great calcium source and a good milk replacement if you're lactose-intolerant (those good bacteria actually lend you a helping hand by digesting some of the lactose for you). It provides between 150 to 400 milligrams of calcium per carton. But yogurt's not the only food to offer a boost from good bacteria. There are dairy supplement drinks, like Dannon's DanActive, a fairly new addition to stores in the United States, acidophilus milk, buttermilk, and kefir, and even tablets that provide a healthy dose of the good bugs.

To complement and reinforce probiotics in your diet, try to include so-called *prebiotics,* which serve as food for the good bacteria in your intestinal tract. Foods that dish up prebiotics include oatmeal, flax, barley, legumes, whole grains, and onions. At least one brand of yogurt, Stonyfield Farm, dishes up both probiotics and prebiotics in the same carton to make sure you get the biggest good bacteria bang for your buck.

Super Supplements

Vitamin (and Mineral) Genie in a Bottle

To save you the hassle of supplement shopping on your own, we've come up with a few branded multivitamin/mineral suggestions. These will pretty much keep you covered for the major vitamins and minerals (except calcium) and the dose is only one tablet a day. (Some supplements look great on the nutrition label, until you see in fine print you have to down two or three a day.) A note for women "of a certain age"—we've got a separate list below that has either less or no iron. Once your periods stop, there's no need for all that extra iron and it could, in fact, be bad for your health. Too much iron in the body can actually damage organs and cause a laundry list of health problems from heart disease to liver problems.

Multi Choices	More Mature Choices
Centrum	Centrum Silver
Kroger Complete Extra	CVS Daily Multiple 50 Plus
Nature's Bounty Women's Exclusive	Eckerd Therapeutic M
Puritan's Pride Multi-Day Plus Minerals	Healthy Idea Therapeutic M
Rite Aid Whole Source	One A Day 50 Plus
Sundown Complete Multi Daily	Safeway Thera Plus
	Theragran-M Advanced

So Many Supplements, So Little Time

We've never taken a count, but it's a cinch that the number of supplements on the market ranges in the thousands, if not tens of thousands. You can choose from vitamins and minerals in any number of combinations and concentrations as well as herbs, amino acids, fatty acids, phytosterols, hormones, flavonoids, enzymes . . . you name it. All without a prescription. It's tough to resist the allure of such a hassle-free approach to improving your health. So, should you dive in and fill your medicine cabinet with supplements? In a word, no. But as with most things in this life, the real deal is slightly more complicated than that. Here's the dish: Pick a supplement, almost any supplement, and we can show you research suggesting that it offers some sort of health benefit. Maybe it's supposed to lower cholesterol, keep your eyesight healthy, lift you out of depression, boost your immune system, help control diabetes, or make weight loss easier. All possible. But the hard reality is that, for most of them, researchers haven't yet hammered out the details—how much, how often, and, perhaps most important, how safe. Our advice? Resist the temptation to buy supplements à la carte and stick with a multi and a calcium supplement for the basics. For everything else, it's on a case-by-case basis. Once you start experimenting with high doses of a variety of unproven supplements and taking them on a daily basis, you're basically delving into complementary medicine—not nutrition—and without a guide. These supplements may be over-the-counter, no prescription required, but they are certainly far from being sugar pills with no chance of potentially dangerous side effects.

Supplement News Central

If you're looking for more info on specific supplements—from cholesterol-lowering products to those that promise to help boost your metabolism and shave off those extra pounds—especially the dish on which ones pass the muster quality-wise, we recommend you check out *www.ConsumerLab.com*. You'll find some of the latest details on which supplements really contain what they say they do, which ones are labeled the way they should be, and which ones are manufactured by the highest supplement standards. All that, plus a primer on the research to back up each supplement's claims.

Desperately Seeking Calcium

Calcium is one mineral that you just can't get enough of from a multivitamin/mineral pill. Vitamin companies can't seem to cram all that calcium into a pill. Maybe for a horse, but not for you and me. And it's tough to get enough from your diet alone, so it's not a bad idea to take a calcium supplement, especially in light of the new info on calcium and your weight. Best calcium deal: Tums Ultra antacid—it provides 400 milligrams of calcium per chewable tablet. The same stuff you get from much pricier calcium supplements. Aim for 1,000 to 1,500 milligrams a day.

Omega-3's for Landlubbers

You can't argue with the research surrounding omega-3 fats—the fats found naturally in fish. There's no doubt that they're good for your heart. Not a fan of fish? There are other ways to get your omega-3's. You can opt for flaxseed, though your body doesn't use the omega-3's it provides nearly as efficiently as it does those that come from the sea. Fish oil supplements are probably the number-one alternative, though just between us, finding just the right combo of DHA and EPA (the two main omega-3's in fish) can be a migraine-producing experience. The American Heart Association recommends 1 gram of EPA and DHA per day, including fish. Okay, so what's the omega-3 count of that fish you ate? Should you get the capsule with 250 milligrams of DHA and 500 milligrams of EPA or should you go for the one that has 500 milligrams of DHA alone, which is not from fish at all, but from algae? We gave up on trying to calculate all that a long time ago. Just dive in and put fish or seafood on your plate twice a week or opt for any one of several brand-name omega-3 supplements that will dish up somewhere in the neighborhood of 1 gram (1,000 milligrams) of omega-3's a day.

Super You!

So, now you know how to supercharge your diet with foods that deliver a winning edge. They're the ones to turn to in order to keep your energy up and your weight down. And when you ask, "What have you done for me lately?" these Superfoods can say "Plenty!"

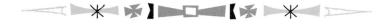

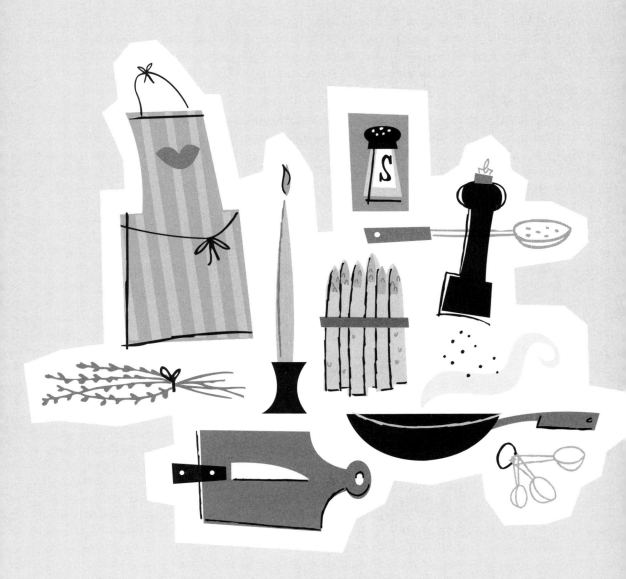

4 The Dish on Eating In

Every once in a while a gal's gotta chill out. Stay close to home. Kick back and relax. But ya still gotta eat, right? So, stick around. We're going to give you the real deal on how to eat in without packing on the pounds. We'll take you on a pantry raid to clear out your cabinets and start fresh. Then, we'll guide you through a makeover of your fridge, freezer and all—what to lose and what to hang on to. And every girl needs a list of staples to always have on hand to throw together a quick and healthy meal. How about advice on the top-ten kitchen utensils you've just gotta have; and a primer on herbs and spices to keep on hand? We'll dish about sweeteners, both natural and artificial. We'll tell you why you might want to upgrade your salt shaker. And lots more! If you've got the "right stuff" on hand, then eating healthy is a cinch.

> Dining is always a great artistic opportunity.
> —Frank Lloyd Wright

The Top-Ten Dish Diva Dream Kitchen Gadgets

A healthy kitchen (that is what we're going for here) is a must for every woman. There are lots of awesome and stylish kitchen gadgets out there that can make eating right a pain-free experience—even for those of us who rank cooking right up there with cleaning the toilets. Here are the top-ten kitchen trinkets we think you won't be able to live without. Sure, you need pots and pans, wooden spoons, and some dish towels, but these are the accessories that make cooking a breeze.

Coffee bean grinder—It's not just for coffee and we all know freshly ground beans are the aromatic best! Use it for flaxseed, one of nature's true Superfoods (because it's a great source of healthy omega-3 oils), so you can add the nutty nuggets to pancakes, muffins, or bake them in bread. Bump and grind as you go, for the freshest taste. These petite machines are also custom made for creating your own spice blends from flavorful whole spices. Make a batch, store it in an airtight container or freeze it, and *voilà!* you've got a flavor supply that will last for months. The next time you want to turn a boring chicken breast into a Dish-worthy entrée, you've got a gourmet spice blend at the ready. French herbal, hot Indian, or Moroccan—take your pick from our spice blend suggestions on page 123.

Rice maker—If it seems unnecessary, then you haven't tried one yet. **Densie Says:** My sister-in-law raved about the wonders of this piece of kitchen equipment for years, before I finally caved and bought one. Best $40 I ever spent. The rice comes out perfect every time—really! You can toss in some saffron, a sprig of fresh tarragon, or a can of chicken broth and it's a great low-cal side dish. Yes, brown rice works too. Just add a tad more water than the directions call for and the cooker automatically adjusts the cooking time. The only downside—most make a minimum of four servings. Try to make any less and it may not be cooked to perfection. But if you live in cramped urban quarters, you may want to opt for a smaller, less expensive rice cooker. It takes up less space and cooks fewer portions.

Mini-food processor—These runt-sized processors make it easy to chop up a batch of onions, bell peppers, celery, coriander, parsley, or shallots, in just the right amount, whether you're cooking for one or for an impromptu celebration for eight. They're more affordable than the big food processors, and they take up less counter space. You'll never go back to the tearful experience of chopping onions by hand.

Bamboo basket steamer—It's the best way to prepare veggies that come out crisp and fresh and not a sickly, army-green pile of mush. It's also a lifesaver for reheating single servings. Better to stick with the larger sizes (they typically come in six, eight, ten, and twelve-inch sizes). That way you can easily fit a dinner plate inside. That's important, because food can stick to the bottom if you lay it directly on the slats. (And it will likely taste and smell a little like bamboo, which isn't usually part of any recipe.)

Two sharp knives—Every girl needs a good, sharp, easy-to-hold medium-size paring knife for peeling, slicing, and cutting fruits and veggies. (Now you've got the pieces to fit in the mini chopper.) And why not be stylish 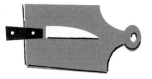 while you're at it? Check out the online Williams-Sonoma catalog *www.williams-sonoma.com* for some really hot-looking blue-, green-, yellow-, and red-handled ones. The other blade you gotta have is a chef's knife, which should be used any time you see the words "chop" or "mince" in a recipe. The shape and weight of this blade make it easier to prep larger quantities more quickly—not to mention less wear and tear on your arm. And just having good knives on hand makes it more likely you're going to prepare fresh produce.

Tongs—How did we ever live without tongs? Put down that kitchen fork! We can't believe how much easier cooking is with these little arm extensions. They're great for flipping foods on the grill, grabbing steamed corn from the pot, turning chicken quickly under the broiler, or maneuvering veggies from pot to plate.

Cutting boards—Throw out the old chipped ones. Nasty bugs can take refuge in those cracks and crevices. Plastic or wood? Makes little difference. Just keep 'em both clean with hot water and soap. Hey, buy a bunch . . . this isn't Wedgewood china! Jazz it up. Make them color-coded—red for meat, green for fruits and veggies. Good idea for food safety too. You don't want the bacteria sometimes lurking in raw meat to make their way into your salad.

Garlic press—Everything tastes better with garlic. Well, almost everything. Our assessment: A garlic press is a girl's best friend. It's an ingenious little gadget that allows you to crush the cloves without scenting your fingers with garlic perfume. You want to flavor your food, not ward off vampires. Buy a good, solid one—the cheap ones wear thin and eventually snap.

Cheese grater—The hand rotary ones. Zyliss, a Swiss company, makes a durable one available in most kitchen stores. **Densie Says:** I have a special one, made in France, that was passed down from my grandmother. It gives me wonderful grated cheese and great memories at the same time. A sprinkle of freshly grated Parmigiano Reggiano on veggies, or salads, or whatever, really adds the edge you're looking for. And these are easier to operate than the stand graters that seem to catch a knuckle or two every once in a while, not to mention the damage it can do to your manicure!

Measuring cups and spoons—Remember, it's all about portion control, baby! Get a set of both liquid and dry (yes, there is a difference, though Williams-Sonoma offers a neat combo cup that lets you accurately measure both—a real plus if your kitchen storage space is in short supply). You'll need a good solid 2-cup Pyrex measuring cup for liquids and a nice set of thick plastic ones for solid measures, ranging from ¼ cup to 1 cup. And don't forget the measuring spoons! A tablespoon is an exact measurement, not the amount that fits into the nearest serving spoon.

Dish Diva Pantry Raid

Let's face it. There are just some items that shouldn't be hanging around in your kitchen, because they're doing nothing for your health and they're taking up valuable space. You might not even like them anymore, kind of like that lime green blouse you had to have but never wore! And they might have expired anyway, like that red plaid blazer you can't believe you ever wore! Open the cabinets and take an honest look. Some of that stuff may have been around so long, you don't even notice it anymore.

They're history! That's the old you. Here, we'll lay it all out for you: What to keep, and what has a big "L" written on the label. Toss those losers out to make room for more healthful basics and ingredients that match your new style of contemporary cooking. The new you takes control of what's in your kitchen. Let the pantry raid begin!

Dish Divas' True Food Confessions: Densie

You never know what you'll find when you start really digging into the depths of your kitchen cabinets. It can be an experience akin to an archaeological dig. Behind the year-old pasta and the canned, marinated artichokes you never used (and dare not remember how long ago you put them there), you might find some entertaining little items. In my last kitchen scavenger hunt, I uncovered, to my surprise, a jar of baby food prunes. Hmmm. A baffling find. No babies either in residence or visiting for quite a while. No secret craving for the stuff. It took a while for me to access my memory banks, but at last, it came to me. The explanation was actually much less interesting than the find itself. I had been experimenting with pureed prunes as a fat substitute. Using baby food prunes is a better alternative than trying to puree prunes yourself. It actually works well in a few foods, like chocolate cakes, gingerbread, cookies, and brownies (and prunes—ahem, I mean dried plums—are awesome sources of disease-fighting phytonutrients). It made me want to try the fat-cutting formula again. With a new jar of baby food, of course. Oh, what's the formula? Try this: Leave out the fat, or keep about one-third of the amount in the recipe and add half the total fat called for in the recipe as prune puree. Confused? If a recipe calls for 1 cup of oil, leave out the oil and replace it with ½ cup of prune puree.

Dish Divas' True Food Confessions: Carolyn

I have no idea where it came from. I really don't remember buying it. But, in my archaeological clean-out-the-pantry dig, I found a can of nacho cheese soup. Was it a gourmet gift gone wrong? Knowing that I wouldn't ever use it, my first impulse was to neatly tuck it away again in the back of the cabinet behind the jars of strange salad dressings and other crazy condiments that would never see the light of day. I just don't have the heart to throw stuff away. It took a visiting longtime gal pal, Jennifer Skiff, to give that kitchen closet a clean sweep. She said, "Go work on your book. I'm going to throw away everything that's expired or looks like a loser. You've got to make room for the good stuff!" Then I let her loose on my clothes closet to purge expired fashions. "Carolyn, I know Hawaiian shirts are back in style, but not this one!" Jennifer did manage to find a cashmere sweater for herself though, explaining, "It's a much better color on me." But she had no interest in the nacho cheese soup.

So, how do you know when it's time to toss the stuff in your kitchen? It depends. Some packaged foods provide clues. Here's the dish on what to dump and when:

When in Doubt, Throw It Out!

. . . .

Even packaged foods are perishable.

"Sell by" Date—the last day the product can be sold in the store, allowing time for its sale and storage. It is more a matter of quality, dictated by the manufacturer, than food safety.

"Best If Used by" Date—the recommended time limit a food should be used for best flavor or quality. It is not a purchase or safety date.

Expiration Date—indicates the last date a food should be used. Eat at your own risk; the food may not be safe.

Longer Lasting, but Not Forever

* Canned foods—beans, fruit, corn, soups, etc.—won't last indefinitely. Toss after about twelve months.

* Dried beans and peas—toss after a year.

* Dried fruits—six months; keep cool in an airtight container.

* Canned fruit juices—nine months, if it's stored in a cool place.

* Instant breakfast packets—six months.

* Ready-to-Eat cereals—six months to a year, if it's kept tightly sealed.

* Coffee (cans)—two years if it's unopened; only two weeks once the lid is gone.

* Honey—twelve months if covered tightly.

* Mustard—two years if unopened; six to eight months if opened.

* Nuts—three months unopened, in a vacuum can; refrigerate after opening.

* Pasta—two years, longer than some marriages, as they say.

* Soup mixes—one year, if kept cool and dry.

* Sugar—2+ years if covered tightly.

* Sweeteners—2+ years.

* Tea bags—eighteen months; refrigeration will make them last even longer.

* White rice—two years if kept in a tightly closed container.

Sweet Talking

Over the years, sugar has been both glorified and vilified. True, it's easy to overdo, and too much of a good thing is always a bad thing. But we can't imagine life without a little sugar on the side. Here's a look at all your sweetest options, both natural and artificial.

Brown sugar—basically just regular white sugar with molasses added for color and flavor. Sold in light and dark shades. Dark has stronger flavor. Brown sugar contains more nutrients than white sugar, but not much. White sugar on the other hand, contains none, even in cup amounts.

Demerara sugar—a granular light brown sugar popular in Britain, but hard to find in the United States. Check out the Internet for mail-order sources.

Maple syrup—made from the sap of the sugar maple tree. Count fifty calories a tablespoon. Look out for fakes. True maple syrup is graded "Fancy" for the best, "Grade A," and "Grade B." If the product label says "pancake syrup," read the fine print; it may not contain any real maple syrup at all.

Muscovado or Barbados sugar—a dark brown sugar with a strong molasses flavor. The crystals are slightly coarser and stickier than regular brown sugar. It's popular in Britain. In the United States, you'll have more luck finding it on the Internet than at the store.

Table sugar—common white sugar or sucrose is derived from sugarcane or sugar beets. Count fifteen calories per teaspoon.

Turbinado sugar—raw sugar that has been steam-cleaned to remove impurities. (True raw sugar is not sold in the United States, because it is not always safe to eat.) It's usually a blond color with a light flavor. You've probably seen packets of it labeled as "Sugar in the Raw," though it is more similar to white sugar than raw sugar.

Pass Me the Honey, Honey

Honey, especially dark honey, provides the same antioxidant punch as many fruits and vegetables. Now, for the first time, researchers from the University of Illinois at Urbana-Champaign have found that people who regularly ate honey (about four tablespoons a day) had more antioxidants in their blood and less artery-clogging damage. Buckwheat and tupelo honeys are among the darkest honeys and were most effective at boosting antioxidant levels. (So, what's the calorie count for all those sweet antioxidants? About twenty-two calories per teaspoon, compared to sugar's fifteen.)

Honey of an Idea

If you like the taste of honey swirled in hot tea or drizzled over baked winter squash, why not explore the world of honey, Honey? The taste of the golden stuff depends on the nectar of the flower the bees buzz by—from orange blossom, raspberry, tupelo, sage blossom, and even spearmint.

Calorie-Free Sugar Imitators

Artificial sweeteners were invented to taste like sugar and save on calories. For instance, every time you choose a diet soft drink instead of the real thing you save 150 calories. So, what's the dish? While artificial sweeteners seem like an easy way to have your cake and eat it too, research has left calorie counters disappointed. It's not clear whether they really help you control your calorie intake and there are lingering health questions. Still, the party line is that artificial sweeteners "are a valuable adjunct to a comprehensive program of balanced diet, exercise, and behavior modifications for losing weight." You'll have to decide for yourself if you're confident about their safety and if using them will make any difference in your weight. A word to the wise: No matter what the ads say, none of them can actually pass the blindfold taste test and pass for sugar. They all have an aftertaste. You try, and decide. Here are the top artificial sweeteners.

Saccharin—The granddaddy of all sweeteners and the most controversial. Probably most familiar as Sweet 'n Low in those little pink packets. Consumer groups are suspicious of saccharin's safety record. There are other options, so we say why take a chance? If you want to avoid it, read labels carefully. Saccharin is sometimes used in a one/two combo with other sweeteners. (Some diet soft drinks use a combination of saccharin and aspartame.)

Neotame—Newest sweetener on the block. Used as an ingredient in food products, but you won't find packets of the sweetener in the supermarket. A whopping seven thousand to thirteen thousand times sweeter than sugar.

Aspartame—Best known as NutraSweet. Though some consumer watchdog groups have advised to either avoid or limit aspartame intake, the FDA, the WHO, and the CDC say it's safe. It's been around for over twenty years and is available in those little blue packets. Most diet soft drinks are sweetened with aspartame. Keep in mind that heat causes aspartame to lose its sweetness, so baking with aspartame is out. Since aspartame can't take the heat, a hot garage where temperatures can reach eighty degrees is not a good place to stash diet sodas. Your best bet is to store aspartame-sweetened drinks in the fridge.

Sucralose—One of the newer sweeteners, approved in 1999. Known as Splenda, it comes in individual packets. Even consumer watchdogs seem to have no major issue with this one. It's actually made from sugar, altered to be six hundred times sweeter. Because this sweetener is heat stable, it's used for baking and to sweeten coffee or tea.

Oh So Sweet, and Natural Too!

If you've decided to give artificial sweeteners the thumbs down, you might want to give the calorie-free, sweet herb stevia (*Stevia rebaudiana*) a try. But don't expect to find it on supermarket shelves along with the other sweeteners. You'll have to look in a health food supermarket in the herbal section, since it's sold as a dietary supplement. But it can be used to sweeten coffee or tea or used for baking. Stevia has a saccharin-like taste, and because it's so sweet, it's easy to use too much. If you're okay with that, then behold the power of stevia:

	⅓ teaspoon powdered stevia extract
1 cup table sugar=	¾ teaspoon liquid stevia extract
	1 tablespoon powdered stevia leaf

Teatime

Always keep tea bags on hand. Green, black, oolong, and even the more exotic white tea are best for providing strong phytonutrients proven to be health promoters. (See chapter 2, The Dish on Diet Basics, and chapter 3, The Dish on Superfoods). But feel free to try herbal teas like chamomile, spearmint, bilberry, or gingerroot. They don't provide the phytonutrients in real tea, but they may offer health benefits all their own.

Instant tea just ain't the same, for taste or health. According to some of our friends at Lipton, instant tea (especially decaf) loses some of its punch during processing and is missing some of the healthy phytonutrients found in regular tea.

Green Tea Taste Test

If green just isn't your cup of tea, because of, shall we say, taste issues, you might want to check out the two green teas rated as "excellent" by the unbiased folks at Consumer Reports. They rated and ranked nineteen green teas for flavor and aroma. The two winners? Tazo China Green Tips (loose or in bags) and TenRen Dragon Well. Just a thought.

Check out our Refrigerator Makeover section for the lowdown on bottled teas. See page 128.

Building a Better Bread Basket

Carolyn Says: Great bread is essential to a great life! I once dragged a couple of college friends into the bread museum outside Lucerne, when we toured Switzerland. There, I found a display of loaves from various nations. The dark breads of Germany, the long loafs of France, the bread sticks of Italy, the flat breads of Armenia. It was the beginning of my fascination with food science. I learned that the reason some breads go stale and hard more quickly than others is because of the type of flour used in baking. So here are some tips for the bread you keep:

Crusty breads—like baguettes, should be eaten the same day you buy them, but to preserve it for more than one day, wrap the bread in both directions in paper or in plastic bags, making sure to seal out all the air first.

Dark, dense breads—whole loaves of pumpernickel or rye often have a really thick crust. Slice only what you need and keep the cut end covered with plastic or foil to seal out the air.

Soft, enriched breads (sandwich bread)—keep them sealed in their packages to stay fresher longer. The same goes for pita bread and tortillas.

Don't store bread in the refrigerator—it dries out, even when packaged in sealed, plastic bags. All breads can be frozen and used later. Freezing halts the staling process. Make sure to seal loaves well in plastic or foil. To thaw, pull the loaf from the freezer at least 2 hours before you need it. Then crisp in a warm oven. It's best not to thaw in the microwave or oven. (Check out chapter 7, The Dish on Entertaining, for more bread tips.)

Branded Fiber Finds

If you make the right choices, breads, crackers, and cereals can provide you with a fabulous dose of fiber each and every day. But as we told you in chapter 2, it's easy to be fooled by high-fiber fakes. We've served up a few examples of high-fiber, whole-grain cereals, crackers, and breads. But don't take this as the holy grail of whole grains. See what fiber surprises you find at your shopping spot, both regular and health food.

(Fiber per serving—Check out the serving size on package labels.)

CEREALS	GRAMS OF FIBER
General Mills Fiber One Bran Cereal	14
Kellogg's All Bran Extra Fiber	13
Kashi Go Lean	10
Post Raisin Bran	8
Health Valley Organic Apple Crunch Bran Cereal	7
Lifestream Flax Plus	5

CRACKERS	GRAMS OF FIBER
Health Valley Original Rice Bran Crackers	6
Ak-mak Stone Ground Sesame Crackers	3.5
Ryvita Flavorful Fiber Whole Grain Crispbread	3
Finn Crisp Caraway	3
Old London Whole Grain Melba Toast	2
Kavli Crispy Onion	2

BREADS

Oroweat 100% Whole Wheat Bread	3
Pepperidge Farm Natural Whole Grain 9-Grain Bread	3
Arnold 100% Whole Wheat Bread	3
Earth Grains 100% Whole Wheat Bread	3
Cobblestone Mill 100% Whole Wheat Hearty Recipe	3

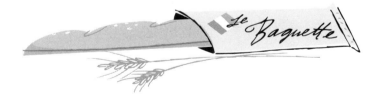

Pastabilities

Did you ever wonder if fresh pasta was better than dried? Well, it's not a matter of superiority. Dried pastas and fresh pastas are built for different dishes. Gourmet Guru Marcella Hazan, author of *Marcella Cucina* (HarperCollins, 1997), is known as the godmother of Italian cooking in America. She says fresh pasta is porous and soaks up too much olive oil, so it's best sauced with butter and cream. Dried semolina pasta, on the other hand, has a harder surface, and works well with olive oil. Marcella poetically observes, "Fresh pasta embraces the sauce; semolina pasta slips it on."

Whole-Grain Pasta Perfect

One of the most neglected sources of whole grains is pasta. Yes, pasta. There are lots of whole-grain pastas from orzo and shells to egg noodles and spaghetti that provide as much as 6 grams of fiber per serving. They're not always front and center in the supermarket, but scout them out. Or ask on your next trip to the health food supermarket.

A *whole-grain pasta* Post-It: There is a definite difference in texture between regular pasta and the whole-grain varieties, just as there is between whole-grain breads and white breads. If it's a new whole-grain adventure for you, the chewier texture may take some getting used to. To keep it familiar, at least in the beginning, try mixing regular pasta and half whole-grain. But don't forget—whole-wheat pasta takes longer to cook, so you'll have to have two pots of boiling water at the ready to cook them separately.

The Dish

The Long and Short of It: Rice

Perfect rice, every time! That's an old advertising slogan for an instant-rice brand. But you can achieve perfection too if you match the right rice to its mealtime mission! Basically, there are different sizes of rice grains and they cook differently.

Long-grain rice (including basmati rice) cooks up fluffy and won't stick—good for side dishes such as pilafs, where you mix rice in with other ingredients, such as nuts or mushrooms or minced herbs.

Medium- to shorter-grain rice is used in dishes such as risotto, paella, and jambalaya. Arborio rice from Italy is the one to stock for making risotto. But many chefs rave about the more expensive Carnaroli variety as the absolute best for risotto.

Short-grain rice has a creamy texture as the grains plump up in cooking and is best used in rice pudding and stuffings. The *shortest-grain rice*, sushi rice, cooks up kind of gluey and is supposed to stick together, so you can pick it up as it supports that slice of raw tuna.

Make a Rice Statement

Want to really up the wow factor on your plate, while you're getting your whole grains? Be adventurous. We suggest you wander off the well-worn white and brown rice path and try varieties of black or red rice, or blends. Some black varieties are as black as ink and as shiny as patent leather, and if it's not simply black on the outside (as some varieties are) it's high in fiber as well. Red rice, which ranges from mahogany to burgundy in color, is a real fiber find, and looks *tres chic* on the plate. But be prepared for sticker shock. They can cost as much as $7.00 a pound.

Check out your local gourmet or specialty food store for these exotic rices. Or order them online. One good source for both red and black rice is *www.farawayfoods.com*.

Gourmet Guru:
Mai Pham

Rice Rules!

Carolyn Says: Shopping for rice in Asian countries such as Vietnam is serious business. While touring the bustling and colorful Ben Thanh food market in Saigon, I turned down an aisle just past the live chickens, and saw dozens of rice varieties displayed in woven baskets. Our guide, Mai Pham, chef and author of *Pleasures of the Vietnamese Table* (HarperCollins, 2001), shared her rice wisdom that day, identifying all of the types. She prefers jasmine rice from Thailand or Vietnam but cautions, "Good rice is fresh-cooked rice. You can start with the best batch of grains but if it's been cooked even a half hour in advance its taste and texture will be less than optimal." Mai also knows a lot about shopping for the best silk in Vietnam!

Can It!

Canned vegetables—Don't listen to the canned vegetable dissenters. While the taste might not be up to fresh standards, the nutrition is pretty darn close. Some vitamins, like C and heat-sensitive B's are partly lost during processing, but total antioxidant levels are sometimes increased by more than 50 percent. How can that be? Heat breaks down the cell walls of the plant, releasing healthful compounds bound inside, making them more available to the body.

Canned beans are an especially convenient item to keep on board. Talk about quick and easy! No soaking or cooking; just open the variety you need and add to the recipe or spice 'em, heat 'em, and eat 'em. Great fiber, good nutrition, and terrific taste and texture on super short notice. But keep an eye out for sodium.

Canned fruit really strays far from the taste of its juicy origins, but it still counts as part of your pound of produce a day. Opt for peaches, pears, mandarin oranges, and pineapple canned in their own juice to keep sugars to a bare minimum. Avoid canned fruits in heavy syrup or light syrup—they'll have more sugar and calories per serving. For more info on canned foods, check out *www.mealtime.org*.

Beans, Peas, and Lentils, Oh My!

Densie Says: When I was growing up in Louisiana, a dish of red beans and rice was standard fare. There was no mention of the healthy side of the bean's character—that they're low in fat, a treasure trove of nutrients, including the B vitamin folacin, magnesium, potassium, copper, and zinc; a rich energy source; and an amazing way to lower cholesterol and manage blood sugar levels. They just tasted good. My, my, how things have changed. Beans are everywhere, from fast-food drive-thrus to the most chic eateries, from the standard, red, white, and black, to the more exotic cranberry, China yellow, and Jacob's cattle. But whatever variety you choose, it's a good choice. And peas and lentils offer a similar outstanding combo of good taste and good nutrition. So, go ahead. Dish up your own hill of beans. We promise it will amount to something.

It's Oil, or Nothing

As we said in chapter 2, The Dish on Diet Basics, your best approach to oils in your diet is to let monounsaturated fats, like olive and canola oils, lead the oil pack, limit saturated fats found in fatty meats and full-fat dairy products, minimize trans fats as much as possible, and let polyunsaturated fats, like soybean and safflower oils, fill in the blanks. No oil is 100 percent mono, poly, or saturated. Rather, they are all an eclectic mix of the three, with one type dominating.

Here's a rundown of the membership roster of some oils you might want to welcome into your diet.

The "Mono" Club

These oils are the highest in monounsaturated fats.

Almond	Hazelnut
Avocado	Olive
Canola	Peanut

The "Poly" Club

These oils are the highest in polyunsaturated fats.

Corn	Soybean
Grapeseed	Walnut
Safflower	Wheatgerm
Sesame	

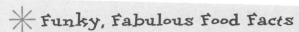
✳ Funky, Fabulous Food Facts

Soybean oil comes from soybeans; peanut oil comes from peanuts; and canola oil comes from the canola plant, but where does safflower oil come from? Safflowers, what else? Never heard of 'em? Well, we weren't too familiar with that bit of botany ourselves, so we checked it out. Safflowers are thistle-like yellow to bright orange flowers that are grown in the Midwest, mainly for—that's right—safflower oil. However, the dried petals can be used as a seasoning. In fact, they're sometimes affectionately referred to as "the poor man's saffron." The oil, however, comes from the seeds of the safflower. Now, aren't you glad you asked?

Olive Oil Vocabulary

Every olive oil has its own unique flavor. In fact, olive oil purists, like wine experts, can taste the difference between olive oils produced in different regions. For example, not only is there a difference between Spanish, Italian, Greek, and French olive oils, their individual flavor characteristics vary from producer to producer and with the variety of olives grown. Usually, the darker the oil, the stronger the olive flavor.

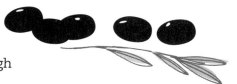

But don't let the dark green glass bottles fool you. While the dark-colored bottle protects the oil from exposure to light, it also makes it tough to check out the real olive hue.

Extra-virgin olive oil—mechanically pressed and produced without the use of chemicals or heat. Best quality you can buy. This is the oil that is made during the first pressing of the olives. It has the most pronounced aromatic flavors, but don't waste them in frying or other high-heat cooking, because the aromas disappear. Instead, savor them in salads or drizzle over dishes at the end of cooking. In Europe, laws require labeling levels of virginity, "extra," "super," "fine" and just "virgin," so look for those words on bottles of imported oils. Store in a cool, dark place to keep that fresh flavor and throw away after a year.

Pure olive oil—a slightly misleading term, pure olive oil is refined with solvents, then those chemicals are "steam-cleaned" away. It's mild in flavor and is better for frying than virgin olive oils. It's often much less expensive and has a longer storage life than virgin olive oils.

Light olive oil—in the good old United States, we tend to shy away from darker olive oils (big mistake) and go for the "light"-colored olive oil, and pay a premium price while we're at it. By the way, "light" on the label here refers only to flavor and color, not to its calorie count. These olive oils are usually in the "pure" category and are best used for frying or other high-heat cooking.

Organic olive oil—meets the requirements for being certified organic. It can still be extra-virgin, but the olives are grown and processed according to organic standards.

✳ The Olive Market

Carolyn Says: As a kid I always liked olives, especially the really big black pitted ones because they fit right on the tips of your fingers—an acceptable way to play with your food. But then I discovered the real culinary wonder of olives. When I was in Morocco, producing a CNN story on the health benefits of Mediterranean cuisines, I toured an olive market in Casablanca. Like a scene from Indiana Jones, we were led by our guide through crowded twisting streets to find an open-air alcove filled with long rows of huge wooden barrels. There must have been over fifty different kinds of olives to choose from, including black, dark green, light green, golden, large ones, small ones, and then special preparations such as olives scented with lemon, spiced with harisa (the Moroccan chile and spice paste) or colorful mixes of various olives. So now every time I see a superselection of olives at a supermarket my mind goes on the road to Morocco.

✳ Olive Oil Observations

Densie Says: I'm a huge fan of olive oil. I actually buy it in three-liter bottles and use it in and on almost everything, from scrambled eggs and hummus to spaghetti sauce and broccoli. I think I must have tried olive oil from almost every olive-oil-producing country around the globe, bought from supermarkets, health food stores, even online organically grown olive oil, until I finally settled on one I really like that hails from Lebanon. I buy it at a local Middle Eastern market. It's dark, it's aromatic, and I can't cook without it. Maybe dark olive oil isn't your thing, but the point is, don't stop with a taste-test sample of one. There are huge differences in the taste of olive oils. Like wine, you just have to find the right vintage that suits your taste buds.

Spice Capades

· ·

They may have said they were looking for gold, but most of the explorers who set out to find the New World were really under royal command to find a shortcut to the spice markets of the Far East. Spices were once more valuable then precious jewels and today they're still the way to adorn dishes with desirable flavors and flair.

There are literally millions of combinations of herbs and spices you can conjure up in your kitchen to give otherwise boring foods a real kick. Your newly invented spice combos may not always work, but when they do . . . you'll wow your friends and family (not to mention your own taste buds) with your culinary acumen. Check out these blends and make them work for you. (Specialized blends are increasingly more available in supermarkets too as spice companies and celebrity chefs create new products based on their customers' internationally inspired palates.)

Be a Global Gourmet

Curry powder—dried red chiles, coriander seeds, mustard seeds, black peppercorns, fenugreek seeds, ginger, turmeric

French herbal blend—thyme, rosemary, basil, tarragon

Herb salt—sea salt, thyme, rosemary, oregano

Hot Indian—cumin, coriander seeds, cardamom, black peppercorns, cloves, mace, bay leaf, cinnamon

Italian seasoning—oregano, marjoram, thyme, rosemary, basil, sage

Jamaican—thyme, cinnamon, ginger, allspice, cloves, garlic, onion

Mexican seasoning—chile peppers, garlic, onion, paprika, cumin, cayenne pepper

Moroccan—black peppercorns, cardamom, mace, nutmeg, allspice, cinnamon, cloves, ginger, turmeric, fennel seeds

Poultry seasoning—sage, thyme, dehydrated onion, marjoram, black peppercorns, celery seeds, cayenne pepper.

Seafood seasoning—dill weed, sesame seeds, lemon zest, basil, tarragon

While whole spices you grind yourself are richer in flavor than dried, these whole nuggets of taste and aroma don't last forever. Their flavor power diminishes over time. The same, of course, holds true for dried herbs. If your dried basil starts tasting like dust, maybe it's time to say bye-bye. A year and a half is pretty much the maximum lifespan of a spice or herb, dried or whole. After that, it loses its kick. Out with the old; in with the new. Or for a perfect solution to this problem, cook enthusiastically with your herbs and spices so you use them up!

Pick a Salt or Pepper

You gotta love it when a gourmet trend goes mainstream, because the prices come down. To get the maximum in taste and convenience, opt for handy one-time-use sea salt or peppercorn grinders. Found in the spice section of the supermarket, several companies (including McCormick and Alessi) are now making these inexpensive "use 'em and lose-'em" jars with built-in grinders. They're light and portable so you can throw them in a briefcase or picnic basket to spice up meals at the office or on the beach. A must-have for fresh pepper flavor or the zing of sea salt wherever you dine!

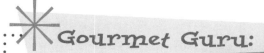
The Lighter Side

Yes, the baron of "Bam!" and "Pork Fat Rules!" was making folks "Happy! Happy!" when I first met him while doing a CNN story on his Creole Light cooking classes in New Orleans in the mid-eighties. As executive chef at Commanders Palace, he was asked by owner Ella Brennan to come up with recipes that lowered her family's risk of heart disease, but didn't lessen the fun. More restaurant customers were craving the same thing, so Emeril added Creole Light dishes to the menu and started a series of packed house cooking classes. The simple origins of "Emeril Live."

At the same time Emeril was itching to create a new style of New Orleans food, moving beyond wonderful but heavy classics such as thickly rouxed gumbos, étouffée, fried fish meunière, and Bananas Foster. So, *new* New Orleans cuisine was born—lighter in fat and brighter in flavor—with Creole seasonings and hot sauces—without forgetting the palate power of a little spicy andouille sausage. He opened Emeril's Restaurant in 1990 and kept on cooking! Sure, he wows diners and the television fans with every drizzle of chocolate and dollop of cream he luxuriously adds to finish a dish, but like all great cooks, he knows how to lighten a creation at a customer's request. And if Emeril can do that with New Orleans cuisine, he's definitely kickin' nutrition up a notch!

Suggested reading: Louisiana Real & Rustic, Emeril Lagasse and Marcelle Bienvenu (Morrow, 1996).

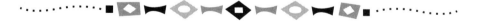

Is Sea Salt Superior?

So, what's the dish on sea salt? Is it really a nutrition miracle from the sea? Well, not exactly. There's not as much difference as you might think. Regular table salt comes from salt mines and is refined to almost pure sodium chloride. Sea salt, on the other hand, comes from evaporated seawater. The crystals left behind are washed, crushed, and dried into . . . almost pure sodium chloride. In other words, both types of salt are about 99.7 percent sodium chloride. While most regular table salt you buy is produced here in the United States, much of the sea salt in stores is imported. Nutritionally, there's not much difference between the two, though chefs we know swear by sea salt's superior taste. Sea salt does contain a few minerals found naturally in seawater, but the amounts are positively minuscule—about 10 milligrams per teaspoon. To get significant amount of minerals from sea salt, you'd have to eat huge quantities. And too much of any kind of salt is not a smart health move. While half of regular table salt contains potassium iodide (a mineral added years ago to prevent iodine deficiency), and all contain one of several additives like magnesium carbonate or silicoaluminate to prevent salt from clumping, several sea salts are additive-free. Still, even some brands of sea salt contain iodine and one of the so-called "anti-clumping" additives to keep the salt flowing freely. Check out the label to be sure.

Upgrade Your Salt Shaker

Carolyn Says: I love cooking with sea salts and have collected them on my travels around the world. As a foodie, I think they taste better. As a registered dietitian, I like them because when you use really good salts, like these, you don't need to use as much to enhance the flavor of your food. To me, there is nothing more wonderful than biting into a July tomato that's been sprinkled with a few crunchy sea salt crystals. And to properly upgrade your salt shaker, you really need to move beyond the shaker and buy one of those salt mills that grind chunks of sea salt. They are just like pepper mills and are often sold in sets.

Salt Shakeup

Even though all salts are . . . well, salty, there is a definite quality difference in types of salt. Sea salt, kosher salt, and other noniodized salts are preferred by chefs who want a cleaner, brighter flavor. Sea salts come from the sea, as their name indicates, and the most prized sea salts come from Brittany, on the coast of France. The sea salts of Brittany are often a light gray color, indicating they have not been processed and still contain minerals from the sea. *Fleur de sel* from Brittany is the ultragourmet choice. The crystals are tinier and more delicate and are harvested off the very top of the sea salt as it dries in the sun. Of course, wherever there's salt water around the world, there can be sea salt. In Hawaii, the sea salt is a reddish color, and is called alae salt. It looks totally elegant sprinkled over grilled fish.

Refrigerator Makeover

Okay, what's in your refrigerator? If your answer is, "A bottle of Chardonnay, two light beers, four kinds of salad dressing, and a few restaurant ketchup packets," then we've got to talk! While it's not necessary to create a scene worthy of "fridge-styles of the rich and famous," what you have on hand will dictate what you'll nosh, especially when you want to eat "*Now!*" So, to help you better stock your cold storage, here are a few ice-box basics.

Want a Cold One?

If you stand there staring into an open fridge, the temperature is going to go up and foods won't last as long. So, as your mom always said, "Shut the refrigerator!" Even when it's shut, the warmest spot is the shelf area on the door, so that's a good place to store relatively long-life things like salad dressings, salsas, and pickles. The coldest spot is near the bottom, that's why the meat drawer is there. The crisper drawer has a higher humidity level to help keep fresh veggies from wilting. So, store things accordingly.

Drinks

Keep **club soda** and **seltzer** in stock at all times. Add your own squeeze of lemon or lime, or buy those already flavored. Just be sure if it's flavored that it's not also sweetened. (It's easy to be fooled.) Avoid those that have high-fructose corn syrup listed as an ingredient; it's just a concentrated, cheap form of sugar. Drink on the rocks or mixed half and half with fruit juice.

Fruit juice—great . . . if you're drinking the real thing. There are so many fruit juice lookalikes out there, it's sometimes tough to tell. The fact is that juice drinks, juice cocktails, and juice beverages are poor imitations. However, an eight-ounce glass of 100 percent real fruit juice, like orange or grapefruit, gives you a healthy dose of vitamins and phytonutrients (and calcium, if you opt for calcium-fortified brands— which we highly recommend). But remember, while fruit juice is great, whole fruit is better. Fruit juice, even with pulp, is low in fiber and, as a result, less able to tame the incessant rumbling in your stomach.

Densie Says: I'm a real fan of V-8 juice. But you haven't lived until you've tried the "spicy and hot" variety. It tingles your taste buds while dishing out a healthy dose of the phytonutrients lycopene and beta-carotene. (And it makes a mean Bloody Mary mix.)

We give our opinion on **diet sodas** in chapter 6, The Dish on Drinks, but we'll say it here too in case you're skipping around. Drink them if you must. Just try not to go overboard. And regular sodas are probably not the best item to keep in stock, though an occasional soft drink won't wreck your healthy eating goals.

What's the word on **bottled teas**, besides the fact that they have some of the snazziest, just-gotta-have-it containers in the store? Should you keep them in your cabinet? Well, despite all the glowing praise we've heaped on tea for being a healthy beverage, bottled teas are a whole 'nother animal. Yes, they contain real tea, and yes, they provide the healthy phytonutrients native to the tea leaf (though not as much as freshly brewed tea). And sometimes they contain small amounts of herbs like ginkgo, ginseng, and guarana. But in addition to all that, you get a whopping injection of calories, mostly from sugar—somewhere in the neighborhood of 150 to 250 calories and as much as seventeen teaspoons of sugar in a twenty-ounce bottle. A word to the wise woman: Read the labels carefully for calorie counts. The calories on the label are listed "per serving." But a "serving" is only eight ounces. If you're just scanning the label for calorie counts as you rush from the refrigerator section to the checkout, you might think your bottled tea provides only seventy calories or so—but that's only for eight ounces. Sorry to burst your bottled tea bubble, but to get the real calorie count for that twenty-ounce bottle, ya gotta do a little mental math and multiply that by two and a half (2.5 x 70 = 175 calories). That's your real calorie count—much more than even a twelve-ounce soda. And you thought you were doing a good thing . . .

Either you're a **milk** drinker or you're not. If you are, go for the lowest fat milk you can deal with for use in cereal, recipes, instant breakfasts, and the like. But it's okay to reserve whole milk for your coffee and tea, if anything less makes you gag. Check out chapter 6, The Dish on Drinks, for more dish on dairy.

Dairy Aisle

Entire books are written about cheese. The French have made eating *fromage* into a fine art. Some New York restaurants even have their very own *maître fromager* to guide customers in their choices. But you don't have to be a cheese whiz to enjoy the cheese of your choice. Nutritionwise, however, we have a surprise. Whether you choose a supermarket brand of Cheddar, a Wisconsin Camembert, or an imported goat cheese, the calories don't vary that much—about 75 to 114 calories per ounce. That gives you more than enough to choose from. But Camembert, feta, Gruyère, and mozzarella fall in the lower end of that calorie range. Keep your favorite *fromage* on hand for a snack with whole-wheat crackers, to dress up a salad, or slice a wedge to have with a crisp Granny Smith apple.

Out with the Mold?

Some cheeses, like blue, Roquefort, Gorgonzola, and Stilton, or the white surface molds on wheels of Brie and Camembert, contain good molds that are essential to their unique textures and flavors. But what about molds that insidiously appear on cheese stored for way too long in the fridge? If you see signs of the fuzzy stuff growing on any soft cheeses, toss the whole package. Those fuzzy mold tentacles easily spread through to cheese parts unseen. For hard cheese with only a spot of green fuzz, you can trim the mold out by cutting off one inch around all sides of the mold, being careful not to let the knife touch it to avoid spreading the mold around. You can cover what's left in clean wrap. Can't stand the thought? If your lip is curled up in disgust, then just toss it.

Yogurt

We've already told you quite a bit about the wonders of yogurt in chapter 3, The Dish on Superfoods, but suffice it to say that it's a healthy addition to your diet because it's loaded with "good bacteria" that may help you fend off disease. But while it's a nutritious food, you'll need to watch out for sugar when you're scanning the ever-expanding yogurt section at the supermarket! It can reach close to eight teaspoons of the sweet stuff in an eight-ounce carton of fruit-on-the-bottom yogurt. And check the "use by" date before you buy and before you eat what's already in the fridge. It could go bad and the number of good bacteria diminishes as the carton gets closer to its end-of-the-line date. If the date's okay, don't panic if you see some liquid sloshing around on the top. It's just the whey separating out. Stir it back in and it'll be fine.

Yogurts generally come in four-ounce, six-ounce, and eight-ounce containers. If you're looking to save calories, go for the smaller containers. And, remember, the more extras it contains, like chocolate chips, granola, or cookie bits, the more fat and calories it's going to provide. Most yogurts are "low-fat" and provide only a few grams of fat per carton, but there are a couple of full-fat yogurts you'll want to avoid for calorie considerations.

Thoroughly Modern Margarines

Margarine choices are multiplying. At the same time, margarines have had a makeover—they're lighter and healthier. All margarines and vegetable oil spreads are cholesterol-free, because they come from plants. (Only animal foods have cholesterol in them.) That makes them better than butter for your heart.

The healthiest margarines are the softer tub or liquid spreads. Because they haven't been hardened by hydrogenation, they are lower in trans fats or completely trans-fat-free. And the ultimate goal is, after all, to choose a spread that's low in saturated fat and trans fats. (For more about bad-for-you trans fats, you can work your way back to chapter 2, The Dish on Diet Basics.)

So, margarine companies have been busy creating newer, better-for-you spreads that still deliver a "buttery taste." Many are lower in fat and calories than butter or regular margarine—which, BTW, are about the same.

But according to Linda Severin, at Fleischmann's, a gal in-the-know about margarines, it's no easy task to please taste buds and meet health demands at the same time. "It's been a real challenge," she says, "to move away from hydrogenated oils, because it changes the texture of the product." Where's the benefit, if you have a spread that's healthy, but it's too soupy? Their latest trans-fat-free spread has managed to add olive oil to the mix, while keeping a buttery taste and texture. We say that sounds like a successful recipe for change.

Cooking Note: Many of the lower-fat, "light" spreads are higher in water and just can't take the heat. We don't suggest you try them for sautéing, because the water will spatter. They are no good for baking either. So, if you decide to cut calories by choosing a "light" margarine, you can use them happily on breads, rolls, potatoes, and cooked veggies. The rest is pretty much a matter of taste. And they vary in taste quite a bit—some are more "buttery" than others, some unsalted, and some a bit sweeter. Stick margarines still exist because, well, people just like them. And they work better for baking, because they act more like butter. Still, the harder the margarine, the more the trans fats, so limit your use of stick margarines to the occasional homebaked treat.

Spread Sheet

. . . .

We did a bit of supermarket sleuthing (disguised as your average shopper) and found a few spreads we can happily recommend as healthful bread spreads.

Light Spreads (forty to fifty calories and about 5 grams of fat per tablespoon)

Fleischmann's Light Margarine
Take Control Light Spread
I Can't Believe It's Not Butter Light Spread
Promise Buttery Light Spread

"Lighter" Spreads (fifty to eighty calories and 5 to 8 grams of fat per tablespoon)

Brummel & Brown Spread with Yogurt
Fleischmann's Premium Blend with Olive Oil
I Can't Believe It's Not Butter Sweet Cream & Calcium Spread
Parkay Spread

Full-Fat Spreads (eighty to a hundred calories and 9 to 11 grams of fat per tablespoon)

Benecol Spread
Fleischmann's Original Spread
Spectrum Naturals Essential Omega Spread
Canoleo Soft Margarine

Carolyn Says: "I remember being with friends at a stylish little restaurant in New York, known for the chef's creative hand, and as we tasted one of the dishes, we found ourselves smacking our lips and asking, "What is that flavor? Is it an herb? Is it the essence of some savory stock?" It was butter! We all had a good laugh and then mourned the fact that we had downed so many dishes broiled dry and splashed with lemon, we had forgotten what a delight butter can be. (I do know that the churned sweet cream butter served with the bread basket at Charlie Palmer's Aureole Restaurant in New York City is so good, I could eat it like cheese.) Butter is, of course, a dairy product, made from cow's milk, and it's pretty much all fat and pretty much all saturated fat at that—the kind that clogs your arteries. It should be used in moderation and savored as you would a fine chocolate. There are terrific gourmet butters to choose from, made by tiny dairies or imported from France or Ireland, where they take their butter quite seriously. Butter comes salted, unsalted, and there are more light versions in the dairy section today. And, if you choose a light one, whipped with some air, you can cut the total fat and calories per tasty teaspoon.

Looking for a Better Butter?

Is organic butter better? Depends on what you mean by better. If you mean fewer calories and less saturated fat, the answer is a resounding no! (We know, it's a butter bummer. It just feels so much better to buy butter from the health food store; how can it not be true?) Butter is butter as far as fat and calories go. But if you're doing your dead-level best to avoid pesticide or chemical residues that are sometimes found in conventionally raised plants and animals, then, yes, organic is the way to go.

Egg Education

Okay, so eggs are high in cholesterol, but for most people that's not a cause to pause. (Check out Cracking the Egg Myth on page 135.) But if you're still in search of a better egg, here are the ABCs of the incredible, edible egg options. Eggs are available for just about every concern, from nutrition and pesticides to animal welfare, and even egg-eating vegetarians. Sometimes egg products address more than one concern, but we've yet to find one that addresses all four. Here's what those specialty eggs are for: *Certified organic* eggs are exactly that—eggs that have been certified organic by a certifying organization. But just because a label says the hens have been fed certified organic grain feed does not mean that the eggs have been certified organic. There are other criteria, such as no use of drugs, which must be met for eggs to be certified as organic.

Free range or *free-roaming* means the eggs come from chickens allowed free access to the outdoors. You'll also see eggs from cage-free hens, which means they aren't confined to a cage, but not necessarily allowed access to outdoor areas. But unless otherwise specified, they may be fed regular grain and treated with antibiotics. Organic eggs and eggs from free-roaming hens tend to be the most expensive.

Vegetarian eggs actually come from hens fed all-vegetarian feed that contains no animal by-products. But they are not certified organic or free range, unless the label says so.

Nutritionally enhanced eggs range from reduced-fat, reduced-cholesterol eggs, to eggs with higher-than-normal levels of vitamin E or heart-healthy omega-3 fatty acids. Egg nutrition is manipulated by changing the hens' diets.

✳ Why do refrigerators have built-in egg holders? You got us. The truth is, that's the quickest way to shorten the shelf life of a carton of eggs. Keep them in their original cardboard or Styrofoam cartons. They'll stay fresh longer. And pay attention to the "sell by" date. It's the best guide for freshness.

What's New, What's True

Cracking the Egg Myth

Repeat after us: *An egg a day is okay.* Once vilified as being the major cause of high cholesterol and shunned by anyone with even a passing interest in their health, eggs have been redeemed—well, sort of. The eggs-heart disease theory has been discounted by experts. But while the facts of the case have been presented and eggs acquitted of any wrongdoing, it seems their bad boy reputation lingers. It's easy to understand why. Eggs are an amazingly concentrated source of cholesterol in your diet (about 213 milligrams each), second only to maybe liver (which has other issues, shall we say), and if your blood cholesterol is high, well, the odds are not exactly in your favor for a long, healthy life.

Here's the dish: If you've already been warned by your doc that your cholesterol is over the top, it might be a good idea to make eggs a some-times thing, just to be on the safe side. However, if your cholesterol is normal and you're not at high risk for heart disease, there's no reason to strictly limit eggs. In fact, that bastion of research and education, Harvard University, found that healthy people with normal cholesterol levels could eat an egg a day without risking their heart health. BTW: Eggs offer several health-promoting nutrients, including vitamins A, B_6, B_{12}, folate, and the phytonutrient lutein.

Perfect Omelet "T'egg-nique"!

If a genie were to grant three wishes to a true food lover, she'd be smart to ask for cooking lessons from the charming and talented Jacques Pépin. Award-winning chef, prolific cookbook author, Public Television cooking-show host, and dean of special programs at the French Culinary Institute in New York, Jacques also counts cooking for three French presidents on his impressive résumé. Most of all, he's a lot of fun and takes care to turn the most complicated recipes into simple steps that lead to your kitchen success. So, you think beating a few eggs into an omelet doesn't rate as haute cuisine? *Mais, non!* As Jacques will tell you, "Egg cookery is one of the most delicate jobs in the kitchen. Technique is imperative to produce the light, fluffy omelets to win you an 'A' in any cooking class." So, follow along with Jacques and enjoy this omelet with fresh herbs from *Jacques Pépin Celebrates* (Knopf, 2001). (You can use one whole egg and three egg whites, if you want to cut down on total cholesterol. Or you can simply share this sizable three-egg omelet with your breakfast companion!)

Suggested reading: Jacques Pépin's memoir with recipes, *The Apprentice: My Life in the Kitchen* (Houghton Mifflin, 2003).

Classic Fines-Herbes Omelet

Jacques Pépin, cookbook author, teacher, and PBS television chef extraordinaire

YIELD: *1 omelet*

3 large eggs

Dash salt and freshly ground black pepper

2 tablespoons fresh herbs (1 tablespoon finely chopped parsley and 1 tablespoon finely chopped mixture of chervil, tarragon, and chives)

1½ teaspoons unsalted butter

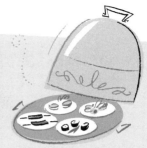

1. For the classic fines-herbes omelet: Using a fork, beat the eggs with the salt, pepper, and herbs in a bowl until well mixed. (When you lift the fork, pieces of egg white should no longer separate from the yolk; the egg should be well homogenized.)

2. Melt the butter in a nonstick skillet 6 to 8 inches in diameter. When it is foaming, add the eggs. Holding your fork flat, so the prongs are parallel to the bottom of the pan, stir the eggs as quickly as you can with one hand while shaking the pan back and forth with the other hand. Continue to shake and stir at the same time, so the eggs coagulate uniformly.

3. When the eggs are lightly set throughout but still moist in the center, incline your pan forward so that most of the eggs gather at the far end of the pan as they continue to set. Now, while the eggs are still moist in the center, stop stirring. You will notice that the mass of eggs has moved toward the far end of the pan; it has thinned out around the edges at the near end. Using your fork, fold this neat, thin edge in toward the center of the omelet, enclosing the thick, moist center. (If the mixture were left to set in one even layer covering the whole bottom of the pan, it would roll up like a jelly roll; thus the center would not be moist.)

4. Press the fold into place, creating a rounded edge. Then run your fork between the edge of the pan and the far edge or lip of the omelet to loosen it. Using the palm of one hand, tap the pan handle gently where it joins the pan to shake the omelet and make it twist and lift onto itself, so the far lip rises above the edge of the other lip. Press with the flat of the fork to shape the omelet into a point at each end.

5. Holding your serving plate in one hand, bang the underside of the pan against the counter at the omelet end, so the omelet moves against the edge of the pan. Then invert the omelet onto a plate, and serve immediately. When cut, the omelet should be very moist, creamy, and wet in the center.

The Lifespan of Your Produce

The road to rotten produce is paved with good intentions. Whether you go to the local farmers' market or are seduced by the awesome display of organic fruits and vegetables at the health food store, it can be hard to resist all that gorgeous produce: The bright red tomatoes, the succulent raspberries, the firm, plump blueberries, and the sweet-smelling melon. But all those mouthwatering fruits and veggies can turn to slimy mush if you don't serve them up in short order. They're not doing your body any good if they're rotting in the produce crisper. And research shows that levels of those health-promoting phytonutrients found in produce drop while the stuff is sitting in your fridge. So eat it while you can. The sooner, the better. Some produce is longer-lived than others, but keep this timetable in mind, before you forget about the stuff stashed in the produce bin.

Apples—tough to spoil, but they can get mealy and tasteless if stored too long. Try to eat them within three to four weeks.

Avocados—don't put them in the fridge. If they're ready to eat when you buy them, they'll be good for only another day or two.

Bananas—keep them out in a bowl; not in the fridge. Really depends on how ripe you like them. If you like them before they've started to show brown spots on the peel, then about three days is it. If you like them very ripe and mushy, then you can hang on to them for about five days. (Then the brown mushy ones can be frozen and used later for baking or making smoothies.)

Bell Peppers—keep them dry and they'll last about a week.

Blueberries—a week to ten days, tops, if you don't wash them in advance. Freeze some for out-of-season blueberry cravings.

Carrots—these are among the most durable of the fruits and vegetables. Will last for about two to four weeks stored in the fridge.

Grapes—keep them dry in the fridge and they can last up to three weeks.

Lettuce—keep it bagged, in the crisper, and you can get good salads for a week or more.

Pears—turn brown easily. But don't toss them just because the peel has brown spots. Slice away the spots and enjoy. Will last in the fridge for two to three days.

Raspberries—one of the most delicate of fruits. Best if you eat them right away, but they can last a day or two in the fridge.

Strawberries—maybe three to four days, if they're fresh when you buy them. Wait until you're about to eat them before washing and removing the stems.

Tomatoes—left outside the fridge away from direct sunlight, they can last two to five days.

Shortcut Salads

You've seen 'em. Those prepackaged Greek, European, and mesclun salads in bags. But you think that somehow, it seems like cheating. What's so hard about chopping up a few salad greens, you tell yourself. That, you can do. But the question is, do you? If you answered no, then give in and indulge in a bag of healthy convenience. How do they stay so fresh? There are no additives. It's a little high-tech magic in the plastic material the salads are packaged in that controls the in and out of gases that cause lettuce to rot. Some even have resealable bags that make them extra convenient. And some are organic to boot. But one word to the wise woman: Despite what the package says about being ready-to-eat, experts say, to be safe, you should wash the greens before you serve them up, just as you would fresh lettuce leaves.

✳ Outside the Box

Some produce just doesn't fare well in the fridge. Avocados, bananas, potatoes, onions, tomatoes, for example. Yes, tomatoes. Ask any foodie and they'll tell you straight away: Keep tomatoes at room temperature to really bring out the flavor and preserve the texture.

Market-Wise

Ode to the Avocado

Are you avoiding avocados because of their over-the-top fatty reputation? Well, don't. As one of the only fatty fruits, it does provide a heftier dose of fat than most other fruits and vegetables (about 5 grams for one-fifth of the whole fruit). But they taste terrific and are a good source of fiber (3 grams for one-fifth of a Florida avocado—the bigger, paler California varieties contain less fat, but they also provide less flavor), healthy monounsaturated fat (3.5 of the 5 grams)—the kind of fat in olive oil—and potassium (240 milligrams for one-fifth avocado). **Densie Says:** I have a sliver almost every evening, when eating at home (and it's in season). You'd be surprised how much taste satisfaction it adds to even the most modest meal.

Should You Go Organic?

Our take on organic? If your Kate Spade pocketbook can handle it, go for it. While organic opponents have been long-winded in their arguments that any pesticide residues on conventionally grown fruits and vegetables are minimal and the nutrition profiles of the two are the same, the findings of a handful of recent studies beg to differ with those arguments. First of all, it's starting to look like organic produce may indeed be more nutritious after all. Organic oranges, for example, have been found to have considerably more vitamin C than conventionally grown oranges. And another study found higher levels of several phytonutrients in organic corn, blackberries, and strawberries, compared to conventionally grown versions. It goes almost without saying that they contain fewer pesticides. That center of independent thought, Consumers Union, recently found pesticide residues in seven times as many conventionally grown fruits and vegetables as in organic versions of the same foods. (Yes, even organic can have some pesticide residues. The stuff is sometimes carried through the air, soil, and water to otherwise organic crops.) Still not sold on the cost of organic? Join a local organic co-op that delivers fresh organic produce weekly. They're often cheaper than the health food store and you can't beat the convenience. Or if you feel like really getting your hands dirty and "living off the land," check for local CSAs (community supported agriculture farms). For a few hours of your time a month you get to eat the fruits of your labor at bargain prices. Some require nothing more than your money and that you pick up your produce on time. Check out *www.nal.usda.gov/afsic/csa/csastate.htm* for a CSA near you.

Another option: Fork over your organic money only for those fruits and vegetables that are most likely to be high in pesticides. One environmental watchdog group fingered these fruits and vegetables as being the highest in pesticide residues. In our book, that makes them the best candidates for converting to organic.

Apples	Nectarines
Bell peppers	Peaches
Celery	Pears
Cherries	Raspberries
Chile peppers	Strawberries
Imported grapes	Tomatoes

Hip & Healthy Heroine:
Deborah Madison

Old McDonald Never Had It So Good

Densie Says: Deborah Madison is a woman on a mission. She's trying to get the word out about the wonderful, uncookie-cutter-like world of farmers' markets. When we spoke recently, she told me about her four market seasons of research, her involvement with her local farmers' market in Santa Fe, and how it all culminated in her writing *Local Flavors: Cooking and Eating from America's Farmers' Markets* (Broadway Books, 2002). Suffice it to say, she knows a thing or two about farmers' markets. "I find it inspiring to cook with foods that are as fresh, flavorful, and exciting as those you find at farmers' markets and that are actually connected to the people who grew them. It means more to me to bring home lettuce grown by local farmer Eremita Campos than it does to buy lettuce grown by some no-name corporation."

Her number-one piece of advice when you make the trek to your local growers' market: Ask questions. Where was it grown? Not all so-called farmers' markets are the real McCoy. Take a taste, if you can. (For some reason, in Texas, and a few other states, it's against the law to sample farmers' market fare before you buy.) And don't be shy to take a taste. If it's not as fresh and flavorful as it looked, just say thanks and walk away. Interact with the local farmers; give feedback. It's part of the experience. Deborah says you simply can't be a passive shopper, as you are in the supermarket. But your involvement will be rewarded with high-quality and intense flavors that, she says, make it easy to keep your cooking efforts simple—and simple, high-quality food pretty much sums up Deborah's philosophy for good cooking, good food, and good health. Simply fabulous!

NOTE: There's no need to frantically search for a farmers' market in your hometown. The USDA has a state-by-state listing at *www.ams.usda.gov/farmersmarkets*

Organic Taste Tests

Carolyn Says: One of the reasons I buy organic produce is because it often tastes better. That's not necessarily because it's grown without the use of pesticides, it's because organic farmers tend to prioritize picking plants that produce better-tasting fruits and vegetables. Commercial farmers with big operations prioritize picking crops that look cosmetically perfect and "travel well" in trucks across long distances. Organic farming is a lot of work and requires more hands-on attention from weeding to careful harvesting. Organic produce may not look perfect, with sometimes odd shapes and a few bug bites, but the big burst of true tomato taste or corn on the cob that brings back memories of childhood makes it worth the trip down the organic aisle.

Organic Guarantees

Only in the last couple of years have organic foods and their labels been regulated. Now, you're guaranteed that if a food says it's organic, it really is. Imagine that! But it only tells you how the food was grown, not about its nutrition. Here's what those labels mean:

100 percent Organic—means the product contains 100 percent organically produced ingredients.

Organic—contains 95 to 100 percent organic ingredients.

Made with Organic Ingredients—contains at least 70 percent organic ingredients.

Densie Says: Forget the way-back-when, hippy-dippy image of organics. It's gone uptown. To learn the latest hip & healthy news in the organic world, I recommend *Organic Style* magazine. It's been pegged as a *Prevention* meets *Town & Country* publication. But the coupling works.

Meat, Poultry, and Fish

If you're a real beef lover, then your absolute best choice would be to choose lean cuts of organic beef (although you will pay a premium for organic products). The cattle are raised without the use of hormones or other drugs and are fed only organic grains with no animal by-products (which, in theory, eliminates the risk of getting mad cow disease) and are certified organic by the USDA. Just remember to keep serving sizes small (about 3 ounces). Even organic prime rib is high in saturated fat. There are also some companies that offer what we call "almost organic." They haven't jumped through all the hoops required by the USDA for organic certification, but they are, shall we say, a cut above conventionally raised beef.

The Lean List

Here's a list of some of the leanest cuts of beef. Since it's the fat in beef that makes it juicy and tender, lean meats can be a bit tough to chew if not cooked properly. It's good to marinate them before grilling or choose a slow-cooking method such as braising to tenderize the meat. But just because they're the leanest doesn't mean you have to limit yourself to these alone. There's still room for the occasional serving of succulent prime rib or juicy rib-eye steaks.

Eye of round
Top round
Round tip
Top sirloin

Bottom round
Top loin
Tenderloin

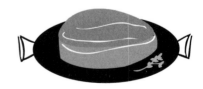

Better Beef Options

Okay. You know that beef labeled as organic is certified by the USDA, but what's with all those organic-sounding terms floating around out there? Here's the dish:

Grass-fed—raised on only grass, though this claim isn't certified or guaranteed.

NOTE: All beef cattle are first raised on grass, then sent to feedlots to fatten up on grain.

Natural—minimally processed without any artificial flavors, colors, or preservatives. Verified by USDA. But—and this is a big one—they are not guaranteed to come from cows raised without hormones or antibiotics.

Free-Farmed—meat and poultry raised in uncramped quarters and without the use of hormones or unnecessary antibiotics. The claim is verified by inspectors.

The Food Alliance Approved—animals were raised on farms that preserve soil and water quality. They are given access to fresh air, pasture grazing, and are given no hormones or unnecessary antibiotics. Claim is verified by nongovernment inspectors.

Chicken Checkup

A recent survey found that up to one half of all chicken is contaminated with bacteria that can make you sick. Salmonella in chicken is a common cause of food poisoning. It won't kill you, but it just might make you wish you were dead. Of course, if you wash your hands and all surfaces that the chicken touches with warm, soapy water, you avoid the possibility of cross-contamination. Also, by using separate cutting boards for meat and produce (remember our color-coding suggestion— red for meat, green for produce) and cook chicken completely (internal temperature of 170 degrees F), even contaminated chicken won't give you problems. Just be aware that the chances are fifty-fifty that the chicken you brought home for dinner is contaminated . . . so, be careful out there. Oh, and BTW, salmonella isn't the only bacteria found lurking in chicken. There are others as well, with such long-winded names as campylobacter, which can pose even bigger problems, because the bacteria are often resistant to antibiotics, making safe-handling procedures even more critical to your good health and anyone else who happens to be sitting at your table.

These Chicks Rule!

Organic, free-range is the healthiest and tastiest choice for chicken. Look for labels that indicate they're raised without hormones or antibiotics. Chickens from these specialty farms often taste better, because the farmers select different breeds and feeds. Most really good restaurants are choosy about their chickens, so call a local chef to ask which regional producers they prefer for tender, great-tasting chicken.

Carolyn Says: I like keeping bags of frozen chicken breasts on hand. They're IQF products, which stands for "individually quick-frozen," so they don't stick together. That way you can grab one or two chicken breasts at a time to prepare a quick meal. Thaw in the microwave, brush on some olive oil, season with salt and pepper, and they cook in less than twenty minutes in a 350-degree F oven.

Go Fish

Fish is a true Superfood. Eating fish, especially fatty fish, like salmon, sardines, and mackerel, has been linked with a lower risk of heart problems, improvement in arthritis and nasty skin conditions like psoriasis. Even the conservative American Heart Association recommends eating fish two to three times a week. But with some fish being in danger of extinction, others swimming in polluted waters, and still others being raised on questionable fish farms, finding the right fish for you can be tough. So, what's the dish on fish? Here are a few suggestions (we don't want to call them rules, because the rules keep changing) to help you make the healthiest fish choices.

* Look for fish certified by *The Marine Stewardship Council*, a guarantee that fish comes from fish farms that are well managed and healthy. (Sold at Whole Foods and Wild Oats.)

* Avoid larger fish, like swordfish, grouper, halibut, shark, or tuna (often used for sushi or tuna steaks). They tend to be contaminated with mercury, an environmental pollutant—something you definitely want to avoid. (However, experts say maybe once a week is probably okay, if you're not pregnant.) For a longer fish list, check out chapter 2, The Dish on Diet Basics.

What about Canned Tuna? The FDA advises women of childbearing years to limit intake of canned tuna to twelve ounces (two regular cans) a week. Tests show that a little more than one out of every twenty cans may contain unsafe levels of mercury. Best choice? "Light" tuna, since it comes from smaller types of tuna than white or albacore tuna—remember the large fish/mercury connection?

* Eat raw fish and shellfish at your own risk. Certainly buy seafood from markets where their food safety standards are high. (First clue: Lots of ice!) Should you eat raw oysters? Food safety experts at the Centers for Disease Control and Prevention like to say sure you can, but it's really a game of Russian roulette. You never know when a bad raw oyster is going to get you. So beware. With sushi, the best places employ specially trained sushi chefs who really know their fish. The first rule of sushi making is demanding the best-quality fish and keeping it clean and cold. But since sushi is by definition raw fish, there's always the risk of contamination from bacteria and other bad bugs, even worms. (Eeeeuuuuu!) Then there's always the possibility of tuna sushi possibly being contaminated with mercury. You may be a sushi fan and never experience a problem, but all it takes is once and, we guarantee, you'll never eat sushi again.

✳ Best all-around fish finds? These fish are your best bets for your health and safety and the least harmful to the environment: abalone, farmed catfish, herring, farmed rainbow trout, wild Alaskan salmon, sardines, farmed sturgeon, farmed striped bass, farmed tilapia, and farmed trout.

Condiment Considerations

"Refrigerate After Opening"—those are the words of warning often found on jarred condiments from sweet pickles to honey mustard. You may have found them on a supermarket shelf and can keep them stored in your pantry, but once they're opened keep them in the fridge to prevent spoilage. And keeping a condiment collection on hand is a great way to gussy up that boring slice of chicken, spice up that beef stir-fry, or dress up your favorite soy burger. Most are okay in the calorie department (they generally range from about ten to thirty calories per tablespoon), with the clear exception of any cream or oil-based condiments, like mayonnaise or tartar sauce. But condiments do have a culinary Achilles' heel: sodium. Even though we're not paranoid about sodium (see what we say about sodium in chapter 2, The Dish on Diet Basics), some condiments really pour on the salt. A few examples for a mere tablespoon serving: chili sauce—230 milligrams; steak sauce—280 milligrams; light soy sauce—560 milligrams; cocktail sauce—1,010 milligrams; soy sauce—1,050 milligrams. Unless you want to make like a blowfish and puff up overnight, you best keep these condiments to a minimum.

Freezer

We've already dispelled a few myths about canned vegetables. What about **frozen vegetables**? Well, they can sometimes best fresh as well. That's because frozen foods hang on to nutrients that are often lost from fresh foods, while they are stored (too long) in the refrigerator. Though we still prefer the taste and texture of fresh over canned or frozen, both are good to have on hand as understudies, when fresh just isn't available. Keep frozen peas, corn, carrots, spinach, broccoli, or green beans on hand for a meal in a minute. Don't forget to keep some frozen fruit on hand too. You can buy frozen peaches, blueberries, or strawberries in bags and use them for making smoothies.

Frozen entrées have come a long way, baby. They're available in an impressive variety of preparations from down home meat loaf dinners to Thai chicken noodle bowls. Some are made to be lower in fat and calories, but all will reveal their nutritional content on the label so you know exactly how much fat and calories you're eating. (Beware of sodium, though!)

Building a Better (Soy) Burger

Here are a few suggestions (feel free to take 'em or leave 'em) for brand names you might want to sample in your search for the perfect soy burger. They're good sources of soy and fine on the fat front. They even offer a decent dose of fiber—something you just can't get from a beef burger. Dish it up on a whole-wheat bun (check the fiber content on the label to be sure it's really whole grain) and you've created a healthy, high-fiber burger. Who wuddah guessed?

Gardenburger Flame Grilled Hamburger Style Soy Patties
Harmony Farms Soy Burger
Morningstar Farms Harvest Burger
Whole Foods 365 Vegan Burger

Densie Says: Keep a box of soy burgers on hand for a healthier version of fast food. Some of them taste surprisingly like the real thing, especially if coupled with lettuce, tomato, and a little ketchup or mustard. Check them out until you find one you like.

There are lots of yummy **frozen organic entrées** to choose from these days, from enchiladas, rice and beans, and Moroccan vegetarian meals to macaroni and cheese and spicy peanut noodles, from brands such as Amy's, Cascadian Farm, and Seeds of Change. They're great to have as a backup when you're just too dog-tired to cook, time is limited (isn't it always?), or you realize when you open the freezer that there is no chicken to make that chicken stir-fry you had on your mental menu.

Should It Stay or Should It Go?

PRODUCT	REFRIGERATION	FREEZER
Fresh Eggs, in shell	3–5 weeks	Don't freeze
Hard-boiled eggs	1 week	Don't freeze
Luncheon meats, opened	3–5 days	1–2 months
Luncheon meats, unopened	2 weeks	1–2 months
Steaks, Roasts, or Chops	3–5 days	4–12 months
Cooked meat and meat casseroles	3–4 days	2–3 months
Chicken or turkey, pieces	1–2 days	9 months
Cooked poultry casseroles	3–4 days	4–6 months
Juices in cartons	3 weeks unopened 7–10 days opened	8–12 months
Hard cheese	6 months, unopened 3–4 weeks, opened	6 months
Soft cheese	1 week	6 months
Margarine	4–5 months	12 months
Butter	1–3 months	6–9 months
Milk	7 days	3 months
Yogurt	7–14 days	1–2 months
Fresh fish	1–2 days	2–3 months
Shellfish	1–2 days	3–6 months
Cooked shellfish	3–4 days	3 months

Source: *www.foodsafety.gov*

Okay, Let's Cook!

You've got the fridge organized and you've purged your pantry. But all this nifty food info does you no good at all if you don't have a clue what to do with it. Do you consider yourself among the cooking-challenged? Not a problem. Cooking is easier than it appears on those cable cooking shows and it's one of the most important survival skills for every health-conscious woman. Knowing how to cook is your secret weapon for good nutrition and good health. (In retrospect, maybe replacing home economics with computer science wasn't such a good idea after all!) Here's a little dish on how to put it all together and make cooking work for you.

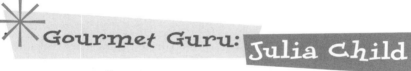

Gourmet Guru: Julia Child

Home Cooks Rule!

Carolyn Says: Julia Child, culinary icon, cookbook author, and the first TV cooking star (her signature "*Bon appétit!*" thrilled audiences way before "Bam!" hit the culinary scene) has always been a champion of home cooks and has encouraged one and all to enter the kitchen with fun as the first goal. Julia visited my home in Atlanta a few years ago for mid-morning coffee and a CNN interview, to talk about her book, *Baking with Julia* (Morrow, 1996). She shared two of the greatest reasons for learning to cook: "When you learn how to cook, you don't have to buy a lot of processed foods that you haven't any idea what's in it." And, she says, "What you make yourself is always better—you aren't trying to save on the ingredients—you use the best, so you can smell and taste the difference. Cooking is a wonderful hobby."

What did I make for Julia when she dropped by?! Believe me, it took some planning. I was a nervous wreck and had the whole staff of Caribou

Coffee in on the fresh ground coffee decision. We picked a smooth rich blend from Kenya. I wanted to bake my mother's recipe for Scottish scones, but knew I'd be in the thick of a TV production too. So, I enlisted the talents of Atlanta chef Scott Peacock to drop by and meet Miss Julia. He was thrilled and made himself at home baking Jessie's Scottish Scones (see page 153).

Julia said she loved the coffee and ate two just-from-the-oven scones. Scott went on to write a cookbook with Edna Lewis, *The Gift of Southern Cooking* (Knopf, 2003). Happy things start in the kitchen!

Suggested reading: Any cookbook by Julia! You may want to start with *The Way to Cook* (Knopf, 1989). More tips from Julia in chapter 7, The Dish on Entertaining.

Recipe Reading 101

Most recipes start with the list of ingredients you'll need and the exact amounts. Though it may seem like a no-brainer, *always* get your ingredients together before you start tossing it all together and cooking. If you don't, you'll get to a point in the recipe where the instructions say, "Now, add the four egg whites, beaten to a soft peak." And you're thinking, "What egg whites?" End of recipe. When you follow the cooking instructions, read through the steps at least once so you know what to expect along the way. We like the recipes that actually number the steps, but if they're not numbered, do it yourself. It's *your* cookbook! Recipe flopped? It may not be your fault, because there are millions of recipes out there that have not been properly tested. That's why major food magazines, from *Bon Appétit* to *Cooking Light,* pride themselves on publishing recipes that have been tested repeatedly, sometime three times, by three different people. Test kitchen cooks (and this is a really neat job!) make sure the instructions are easy to read and the recipe will in fact turn out just like the photograph.

Jessie's Scottish Scones

Jessie Robertson O'Neil, Carolyn's Scottish mother

YIELD: *12 scones*

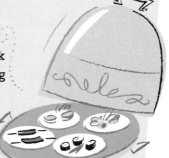

1½ cups all-purpose flour

2½ teaspoons baking powder

2 tablespoons sugar

¼ teaspoon salt

3 tablespoons butter, stick margarine or shortening

½ to ⅔ cup milk

1 egg, slightly beaten

1 Preheat the oven to 400 degrees F.

2 Grease and flour a baking sheet; set aside.

3 Stir the flour, baking powder, sugar, and salt together in a bowl. Cut in the butter with a pastry blender until it resembles coarse meal.

4 Whisk ½ cup milk with the egg in a small bowl.

5 Form a well in the dry ingredients. Add the milk mixture to the dry ingredients and stir just until crumbled. If too dry, add the remaining milk. Be careful not to overwork the dough.

6 Transfer the dough to a lightly floured work surface. Cut into two pieces. Form each piece into a round, ¾-inch thick. Cut each round into six triangles.

7 Place the triangles 1 inch apart on baking sheet. Bake 15 to 18 minutes or until golden brown.

NOTE: For a savory variation, add 1 cup Cheddar cheese, ⅓ cup green onions, 1 teaspoon powdered mustard, and ¼ teaspoon dried marjoram.

Secret (Cooking) Agents

Great cooks and professional chefs have learned a few tricks along the way to make their food taste great. Sure, it's easy to add another chunk of butter to the sauce, but the following tips add flavor without additional fat. And like any magic ingredient, if you add too much, you'll break the spell! We asked Chef Kevin Rathbun, owner of Rathbun's, for his secret agents in the kitchen. He created menus for many popular Atlanta restaurants, including Nava, Blue Pointe, and Buckhead Diner. And Kevin not only likes cooking healthy dishes with lots of flavors, he lives it! Over the past two years, he's successfully dropped the extra pounds that tend to jump onto a chef's body by adding basketball workouts to fight kitchen stress and cutting way back on "tasting everything" he cooks.

Salt: Kevin believes salt is the key ingredient in cooking. "It brightens up your food." But you've got to know when and how to use it. Added to cooking water for pasta or potatoes or in soups or stews, the salty flavor will be more intense as the liquids cook down. So go easy along the way.

Carolyn Says: I believe for both taste and health, salt is best *added* to foods—from eggs to salads—right before you serve them. A last-minute sprinkling from your salt mill will add that crunch and give more of a "flavor hit." You get the salty satisfaction, with the least amount of salt.

Dried Herbs: Yes, certain dried herbs, such as oregano and bay leaves, are much more potent than fresh. (Remember to remove whole bay leaves from dishes before serving.) Kevin says, "Dried herbs have a completely different flavor and add complexity to stocks and sauces."

Turn Up the Heat: Kevin, who's originally from Texas, is a self-proclaimed chile fanatic. But that doesn't mean foods have to be so hot you scream! "At Rathbun's, my dishes are never over-the-top hot. Chiles should add flavor and heat, but you should still be able to taste the food."

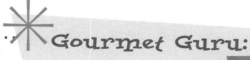

Gourmet Guru:
Shirley Corriher

Food Science Secrets

Sure, cooking is an art, but there's quite a bit of science that explains why recipes work . . . or not. One of the best at explaining the how's and why's of cooking is Shirley Corriher, author of *Cookwise* (Morrow, 1997). Ask Shirley why toast turns brown and lobsters turn red and she'll solve the mystery right down to the last molecule. Her advice: "Spot mistakes before they happen, so you don't waste time and ingredients." Shirley says most beginning cooks ask, "How do you tell when it's done?" Her advice is threefold—use your sense of touch to see if baked goods spring back; use your sense of taste to see if vegetables are tender, and use a meat thermometer to see if meats are cooked to proper internal temperatures. "Just don't keep opening the oven door to check over and over! Every time you open the oven door, the temperature plunges by a hundred degrees. Be patient, and have confidence in your kitchen!"

How Safe Is Your Kitchen?

They say that safety starts at home and that's especially true with food safety. You don't want salmonella and E. coli invading your dream kitchen. Food-borne illness can be a serious issue with complicated, even deadly side effects, but the rules for keeping your kitchen clean and safe are really pretty simple.

1   Wash your hands before, during, and after food preparation. The American Dietetic Association and Con Agra Foods did a survey and found that over 50 percent of people don't wash their hands when they cook! Gag me with a spoon! Hand washing kills germs if you use warm soapy water and wash for at least twenty seconds. Did you just lean over and pet the dog? Wash your hands again!

2   Keep ready-to-eat foods and raw meats away from each other! Use our color-coded cutting board system to keep track—green for veggies, red for meats. You don't want to cut up raw chicken

for the cookout and then slice the cabbage for the coleslaw on the same cutting board. And remember to wash utensils and plates used for raw meats and fish before using them for anything else. One big fat cookout mistake: Taking raw meats to the grill on a platter, then placing the cooked meats back on that same platter without washing it. Those raw juices can contaminate your sirloin and totally ruin your cookout!

ALSO: Use a paper towel, not a sponge, to mop up raw meat juices so you can just throw it away after cleaning the counter.

3 Cook meats to proper temperatures. The only really reliable way to do this is with a meat thermometer. Not only will meats be safe to eat, they'll taste better if they're not overcooked or undercooked. Hamburgers should be cooked to 160 degrees F and poultry to 170 degrees F. Can't remember? Most meat thermometers have proper cooking temps written right on them. Or go to *www.homefoodsafety.org* for a handy chart.

4 Refrigerate foods pronto, to below 40 degrees F. Whether it's leftovers from dinner or the foods on your cookout buffet, you shouldn't leave them out at room temperature for more than two hours. If you're outside and it's hotter than 90 degrees, you shouldn't leave them out any longer than one hour. Bad bacteria love warm temperatures—so give them the big chill!

The Heat Is On!

With some help from Gourmet Guru Shirley, here's how to turn up the heat and start cooking. May the best pan win!

Steaming—Hotter than boiling, because steam is over 500 degrees F! Great for quick cooking of vegetables to keep nutrients alive. But leave green veggies in the steam too long (over 7 minutes) and they'll lose their pretty, bright green color.

Boiling—Water boils at 212 degrees F, and the temperature will stay the same when you boil foods. But make sure the water is at a full boil before tossing vegetables in to minimize loss of water-soluble vitamins and lock in flavors. Sometimes you want the flavors to end up in the water, as in making stocks where you boil celery, carrots, onions, and meat bones, for example, and then simmer for a long time to create a super tasty liquid.

Poaching—Perfect cooking method for eggs, chicken, or delicate fish. Keep the liquid just below a simmer and follow poaching times recommended in the recipe.

Braising/Stewing—Long, slow cooking is great to tenderize lean cuts of meat. Braising adds lots of flavor when the braising liquid contains wine and is seasoned with aromatic herbs and spices.

Sautéing/Stir-frying—Both of these methods require just a small amount of fat in really hot pans and require you to pay attention and move the foods around rapidly. The word sauté comes from the French verb "to jump," so keep the foods flipping. That's why sauté pans have those long handles and wok cooking employs large utensils to toss the food.

Avoid PAN-ic

To successfully sauté meats, such as sliced boneless skinless chicken breasts, Gourmet Guru Shirley Corriher says get the pan hot first, add your oil, swirl it around to warm it up, and then add the chicken. "Stay calm. The chicken pieces will stick to the pan. This is okay. Have a Zen moment of patience." Don't chisel away at the meat trying to move it. It will take a full minute for the chicken to sear and brown and release itself from the pan. Then you can start moving it around. Brown the first side, flip it over, and brown the other side until the breast is firm to the touch, juices run clear, and a meat thermometer reads 170 degrees F.

Grilling—Whether you choose a gas grill or real live hot coals, grilling demands you never leave your post. (That's the kind of cooking dedication guys are drawn to—or is it the requisite beer in the other hand?) Grilling is a great low-fat cooking method because the fat drips out of the meat and the juices are sealed inside. (See chapter 7, The Dish on Entertaining, for more hot grilling tips.)

Baking—Remember the Easy Bake Oven? All that fun with a lightbulb and those teeny, tiny pans. Well, of all the cooking methods, big-time baking can be the most challenging and frustrating, but also the most rewarding. Huge books are written about bread baking and cake baking and pastry arts. You may be able to wing it with stir-fry, tossing in ingredients that inspire you at the moment, but baking requires a steady commitment to the recipe. One extra spoon of baking powder or one forgotten egg white and you and your cake will fall flat. Follow the directions, sister!

Roasting—Two words of advice here—meat thermometer! Perfectly roasted meats, from succulent chickens to mouthwatering rib roasts, to that intimidating bird at Thanksgiving, all require you use the proper temperature for the proper length of time.

Frying—Yummy? Yes. Off limits? No. Read on and you'll learn how to fix your frying.

Straighten Up and Fry Right

Even though fried foods are on the "go-easy" list for gals concerned about fat and calories, there is a big difference in how greasy (and therefore, how calorie-filled) fried foods are. It all depends on how they are prepared. Basically, the hotter and fresher the frying oil, the lower the amount of total fat that will end up in the food. Peanut oil, olive oil, canola oil, and safflower oil have the highest smoke points (the temperature at which the oil starts to smoke and break down), so they are great choices for deep-fat frying. (NOTE: Extra-virgin olive oil has a lower smoke point so don't use it for deep-fat frying.) That's why a thermometer is crucial for frying right—you can see when the oil gets to the optimal temp. For big pieces of food, like chicken, the oil should be 350 degrees F. For smaller pieces, like French fries, the oil should be hotter—at about 375 to 390 degrees F. If you've fried it right, the oil stays on the outside of the foods, where the surface is browned and crispy. The inside is cooked to perfection from the heat, not from penetration of the oil.

Gourmet Guru: Mary Risley

Accessorize Your Breasts

Sometimes cooking dinner means pulling out a basic recipe and dressing it up, depending on your cravings or the setting. It's not unlike the simplicity of that little black dress—cute with sandals at the beach—demure with pearls at the theater—or sexy with high heels and dangly earrings for a night on the town. So, let's take the entrée version of that *LBD,* the boneless, skinless, naked chicken breast, and accessorize it to entertain the many moods of your taste buds. To help guide us through this food and fashion, we turn to Gourmet Guru Mary Risley, founder of Tante Marie's Cooking School in San Francisco and author of *The Tante Marie's Cooking School Cookbook* (Simon & Schuster, 2003). Mary has coaxed thousands of novice cooks closer to the stove through her hands-on classes. "These are really smart people who excel in their careers making money in medicine, law, or financial companies, but they come to me because they never learned to cook!" Mary likes our idea of teaching a simple but important skill—sautéing a chicken breast—and then encouraging creativity in various presentations. So, on with the show.

A Simple Chicken Breast Sauté

Mary Risley, Tante Marie's Cooking School, San Francisco

1. Remove the excess fat and sinew from two boneless, skinless chicken breasts.

2. Place shiny side down on a cutting board and cover the breasts with sheet of wax paper.

3. Pound the breasts with a wooden kitchen mallet or a rolling pin to even the thickness.

4. Season with salt and pepper.

5. Heat a medium-size sauté pan and add enough oil to lightly coat the bottom.

6. Add the chicken breasts, without crowding the pan.

7. When a half inch of white shows on the sides of each breast, turn them over with tongs.

8. Cook until firm to the touch and the juices run clear.

9. Set the chicken aside on clean plate.

After sautéing the chicken breasts and setting aside, now it's time to accessorize! Each of these recipes is for two chicken breasts.

Lemon Caper Chicken—Deglaze the pan with white wine, add rinsed capers, very thin slices of lemon, and minced parsley. Add chicken breasts back to the pan to warm in the sauce and serve with orzo pasta.

Tomato Garlic Chicken—Add chopped garlic, chopped tomato, tomato paste, and red wine vinegar to the pan. Place the chicken breasts back in the pan to warm with the sauce and serve with roasted new potatoes.

Taste of Thai Chicken—Stir in sliced scallions and sliced shiitake mushrooms, remove from the pan and stir in tamari sauce (a slightly thicker soy sauce), rice wine vinegar, and a teaspoon of peanut butter. Add the scallions and mushrooms back to the pan and the chicken breasts to warm. Serve with steamed brown rice.

Green Chile Chicken—Deglaze the pan with chicken broth, add chopped scallions, minced jalapeños, long thin slivers of mild green chiles (such as poblano). OPTIONAL: Whisk in ¼ cup of light cream to finish the sauce. Add the chicken back to the pan to warm with the sauce and serve with black beans and rice.

But I Don't Want to Cook!

Sometimes you want to eat at home, but you don't want to cook at home. *Voilà!* That's when you pick up the phone and order in. But don't fall into the extra-large pizza trap or the Chinese-dripping-with-oil habit. It is impressive how many restaurants are ready to serve via carry out and home delivery. When you visit restaurants you like, make sure to pick up one of their carry-out menus and keep them on file at home. And to order a healthy, well-balanced meal from those menus, the same restaurant rules apply as those we'll talk about in chapter 5, The Dish on Eating Out. One advantage of eating restaurant foods at home is that you can add a personal touch from your spice cabinet and your plastic containers are right there ready to store extra-large portions as leftovers.

The Dish on Eating In   161

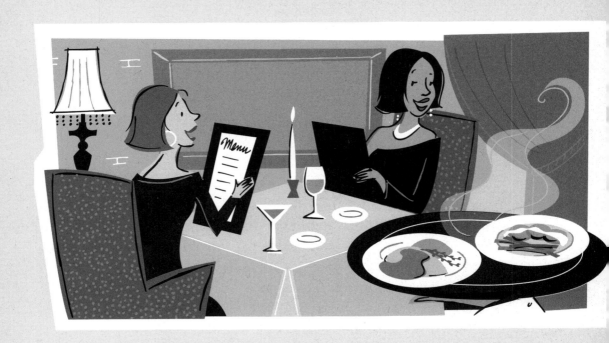

5 The Dish on Eating Out

"**Check, please**" are two of the most fattening words in the English language, says a friend of ours, Larry Lindner, a writer for the *Washington Post*. But, we say, it's not a *fait accompli*. Dining out doesn't always have to mean pigging out! It's simply a matter of making the healthiest choices. And stylish women like you eat out a lot! To help, we turned to our friends in the culinary world to guide you toward the dishes that will keep you looking fabulous and away from those that won't. We'll give you tips on working with your waiter to get what you really want. "Hello, my name is Chad and I'll be your server this evening." Chad can be a big help if you know the right questions to ask. You'll also find suggestions and some recipes from our Gourmet Gurus (top chefs and food pros) who've put their kitchen creativity into overdrive to wow customers with great-tasting culinary delights that, by the way, are easy on the waistline. We'll even introduce you to our own personal

> One cannot think well, love well or sleep well, if one has not dined well.
> —Virginia Woolf

Hip and Healthy Heroes and Heroines—awesome insiders who manage to stay slim and trim even in the midst of dining pleasure and temptations. And we don't ignore the reality that even dishy women resort to fast food and takeout in their fast-track lives every once in a while. So, we'll tell you how to grab and go without the guilt.

Eating Out Is Definitely In

Add this to your "to-do" list: Develop survival skills for eating out. That's a must, because what used to be a special-occasion splurge is now just a regular part of everyday life. According to the National Restaurant Association (a group that knows a thing or two about people who would rather make reservations than make dinner), about half of all the food bucks we spend goes to meals eaten out, and surveys say we eat out a lot—at least four times a week. So, the old notion of throwing calorie caution to the wind when you are holding a fork and knife in a restaurant—because you don't eat out that often—just doesn't cut it anymore. Those calories not only count, they are adding up faster than ever. (Think finance charges on your credit card!) But since you're not about to give up your favorite Italian trattoria for lunch or that lovely little Thai place for dinner, the key is learning how to decode menus so that you can dine in style and good health. And since active lifestyles today often mean living off the land, we'll help you find the best of the bunch along fast-food lane if that's where your wheels are turning.

Restaurant Savvy 101

At an evening cooking class on healthy eating at the Cook's Warehouse in Atlanta, instructor Maureen Petrosky, a petite and perky thirty-something chef and wine expert (trained to handle a whisk and a wine opener with equal aplomb), prepared grilled fish with a pineapple mango salsa, as the conversation turned to restaurant survival skills.

"If the menu says pan-seared, it can actually be cooked in a lot of butter. Ask them to grill it," Petrosky advised.

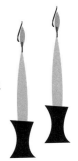

One young woman attending the class, said she cuts temptation off at the pass. "I enjoy the portion I think is sensible and then pour red pepper flakes, or salt or whatever, over what's left on the plate so I won't be tempted to eat the whole thing." (Okay, so we'll put that in the category of whatever works for you!)

A couple in the class said they always ask to split the entrée and tell the waiter they will tip a little more for this special service. That's using the ol' noodle! Another woman, who prefers to enjoy two appetizer courses for dinner rather than an entrée, is adamant about sticking with what works for her. "I refuse to get trapped into the expected pattern of ordering appetizer, entrée, and dessert. I order what I want."

All seemed to agree that restaurant-portion sizes are out of control these days. Our solution? Become the carry-out queen and warn your server ahead of time you'll need a doggy bag.

*Enlist the waiter's help by striking a deal. "You help us to eat less, and we'll tip you more." Bigger tips—smaller hips!

Portion-Size Sins

Portion distortion. Out-of-control portion control. Whatever you call it, we have a problem here. While the nutrition feds (USDA and FDA) say a serving size for a bagel, for example, is two ounces, your average deli-sized bagel is more like 5 to 6 ounces. And while the government calls 8 ounces a serving size for cola, you'd be hard-pressed to find that size anywhere. At fast-food restaurants, soft drinks have swollen to an average 23 ounces, though it can go as high as 42 ounces, if you "biggiesize it" (and you'll be jolted with a shocking 530 calories and 126 milligrams of caffeine). Ask for fries and you're cajoled to "supersize those fries" for only pennies more. Where are all those extra calories going? Right where you think they're going. Order a few of these monstrosities and you'll be biggiesizing way more than you bargained for!

And the bigger the portion size, the more you eat. Researchers have actually taken the time to study this fattening phenomenon and yes, it's true. You see more, you eat more. We mere mortals don't seem to have an inner monitor that tells us to eat less when we're served more. We tend to just keep shoveling it in.

This growing problem is being watched closely by critics. Not much gets by the eagle eye of Nancy Young, Ph.D., R.D., of New York University, who's been taking restaurant-portion sizes to task for almost a decade. We like to think of her as the patron saint of portion sizes. She says she has profiled three degrees of portion distortion. *First degree,* or the least damaging, are fine dining restaurants—the more expensive the restaurant, the less likely you are to encounter out-of-control portion sizes. (Though even this doesn't hold true 100 percent of the time. The most expensive burger in New York City, a $41 Kobe beef burger, contains a record-breaking 20 ounces of beef!) *Second degree* damage, believe it or not, goes to fast-food chains. While they do supersize, at least they make it crystal clear that you're getting the extra-extra-large ahead of time. The *third degree,* and winner for the most over-the-top portion sizes, according to Young, is reserved for casual dining restaurant chains. There's no warning that they're going to pile the plate as high as an elephant's eye, but that's part of the show! These mid-priced family restaurants actually pride themselves on the gargantuan serving sizes they dish up for hungry guests. Of course, the often hour-plus wait for a table at these restaurants indicates they must be doing something right when it comes to customer satisfaction. America loves a bargain.

You Have the Right to Remain Healthy: Don't Be Shy about Asking for What You Want

Remember, you can ask for what you want, because restaurants are in business to serve you and keep you coming back to fill those seats. "I listen to customers," says chef Tommy Klauber of the Colony Beach and Tennis Resort in Long Boat Key, Florida. When more diet-conscious diners started asking to split salads and get smaller portions, he created "Little Dishes to Share."

This refreshing "can-do" attitude in restaurant customer service is good news, especially for the menu-reading challenged among us, who need help choosing healthier dishes. Menus that warn "no substitutions" are out of style. If a restaurant refuses to comply with your requests, find someplace else that will. It's all about service!

Think about it: Restaurant meals are, on average, 20 percent fattier than home-cooked meals.

—USDA

These days, 56 percent of people say they find it hard to eat healthy foods when they eat out. That's up from 44 percent in 1990. Apparently, it's not just a matter of asking for salad dressing on the side.

Source: *Health Focus International Trend Reports*

Gourmet Guru: Danny Meyer

Halve It Your Way

"You shouldn't have to be Sherlock Holmes to sleuth out light choices," says Danny Meyer, owner of New York's popular Union Square Café. Meyer, who is on a mission to promote hospitality in the hospitality industry (what a concept!), not only encourages chefs to create lighter dishes, he trains the wait staff to recognize them. "Our waiters know about the menu and are proud of their knowledge, so guests can feel comfortable asking for suggestions." Meyer, who also owns New York's Gramercy Tavern, Tabla, and 11 Madison Park, suggests a new customer service slogan: "Halve it your way." He wants to let diners know it's just fine to order appetizer portions if they're counting calories. It's all a part of what he refers to as the Restaurant Patrons Bill of Rights, including the right to substitute lower-calorie side dishes. Danny says, "If the halibut comes with mashed potatoes, but they'd rather have the boiled potatoes from another dish, then that's okay."

Navigating the Menu

Okay. Reality check. It's time to get savvy about ordering from the menu. First, you'll need a quickie course in modern menu-speak, so you'll know how to maneuver the sometimes mind-bending maze of options when Chad and company come to take your order.

You might already have guessed that "crispy" can be a code word for fried. And "creamy" a red flag that butter is lurking. But did you know that "poached" isn't always the light way to go? Some chefs actually poach seafood in butter or oil (OMG!), not the usual water-based broths. That doesn't mean you can't enjoy the occasional tempura-battered fried shrimp or side of creamed spinach. It just means that when you see them on the menu, you know it's time to take pause. You can choose to either limit portions, or limit the number of times you order these higher fat choices.

Rather than viewing restaurants as minefields full of fat and calories that make it impossible to fit into that chic little number you bought to wear to dinner—we are pleased as planter's punch to report from the restaurant trenches that many chefs today are extending a helping hand to guide you to healthy menu options. We feel better already.

Who Turned Out the Lights?

While chefs may be dishing out healthier fare, few menus highlight the dishes that are lower in fat and calories. While promoting lighter dishes was all the rage in the early 1990s and restaurants boasted about an alternative Spa Cuisine menu or used little hearts to draw attention to light dishes, this special billing was short-lived. Nobody wanted to be the only killjoy at the table ordering the diet plate. And too many diners assumed "healthy" meant flavorless and unappealing, so the trend went the way of the now extinct McLean burger. (FYI: McDonald's low-fat burger experiment used seaweed as a key fat-saving ingredient. Customers didn't bite.) As Linda Gilbert, president of Health Focus, found out in numerous consumer surveys, "No fat, no salt, no sugar, no flavor, no customers."

Today, lighter menu choices are still there, but they are blended in with the rest of the menu. Healthy dishes such as gazpacho, grilled chicken, and pasta primavera have become part of mainstream dining. You just have to know who the good guys are. And you don't have to settle for less fun, because now chefs borrow interesting ingredients from Asian and Mediterranean cuisines to add bold flavors to dishes without adding more fat. So, thanks to globe-hopping chefs, these lighter dishes taste better than ever!

You'd Better Learn the Lingo

Chef Mark Erickson, vice president of Continuing Education for the Culinary Institute of America, suggests to really be on top of your game, you should become fluent in menu-speak by taking the time to learn more about culinary techniques and terminology. That way you can ask, "What is it sauced with?" A beurre blanc is high in fat. A coulis of vegetables is not.

To Beurre, or Not to Beurre

Tomato Beurre Blanc—154 calories for 2 tablespoons (butter sauce, flavored with tomato)

Tomato Coulis—30 calories for 2 tablespoons (pureed tomato, flavored with a little olive oil, chicken stock, maybe garlic and herbs)

MENU-SPEAK MADE EASY

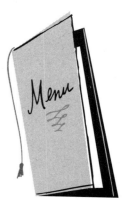

Fat by Any Other Name . . .

Aioli—translation: mayonnaise with garlic

Bard—to lace with fat, insert pieces of fat in a leaner meat

Beurre—butter's French name

Béarnaise, Maltaise, etc.—watch the "-aise," which indicates egg-based mayonnaise

Béchamel—a cream sauce prepared with a roux (a mixture of equal parts flour and butter)

Bisque—most often a cream-based soup

Crispy—code word for fried!

Crispy-seared—another clue oil or butter was used to crisp the outside

Crusted or Encrusted—coated with nuts, bread crumbs, or potato, pan-fried until crispy

Fritto Misto—pieces fried

Frizzled—often onions or leeks are deep-fried until crispy

Pan-Fried—may as well be deep-fat fried

Silky—if a sauce is described as "silky" it's usually finished with cream or butter

Vol-au-vent—in a butter-laden puff pastry shell

Leaning Toward Leaner . . .

Au Jus—pan juices often reduced with no fat added

Braise—slow-cooked to tenderize meats or fish, often little added fat

Brodo—Italian for "broth"

Broth—fragrant water-based sauce with infused flavors; i.e., chicken and lemongrass broth

Coulis—all hail the coulis, often a no-fat-added puree of vegetables or fruit

Flame-seared—indicates grilled over open fire, fats can drain off

Fumet—a fish stock

Medallion—meat that is cut into small rounds (a good thing if looking for small portions)

Pan-Roasted—often pan seared in butter or oil, then placed in oven to roast

Provençale—South of France–style sauce with tomato and other vegetables

Relish—savory mix of fruits and/or vegetables

Salsa—the classic is with fresh tomatoes, onion, cilantro, and chiles, but can be made with fruit and even black beans too

Ask Questions If It Says:

Grilled—watch out for butter or oil slathered on during grilling

Nage—a broth or fumet infused with small amounts of butter

Roasted—watch out for extra fat used in roasting: i.e., butter basted on roasted chicken

Poached—not always in water, watch out for poached in oil or butter

Sautéed—butter or oil are used, chefs can limit amount if asked

Steamed—watch out for butter or oil added after the steaming

Densie Says: Check out *Food Lover's Companion* by Sharon Tyler Herbst (Barron's, 2001). You'll find answers to your questions regarding nearly six thousand food, drink, and culinary terms, from *au jus* to *zuppa*.

CIA Secrets (the other CIA!)

Think chefs are clueless about nutrition? *Au contraire!* Chefs in training at the Culinary Institute of America in Hyde Park, New York, spend part of their extensive schooling (which includes everything from ice carving to icing on the cake) at the St. Andrew's Café, where contemporary menus blend good taste with good health. Chef Mark Erickson helped shape the CIA curriculum. "It is a critical part of our training process that chefs learn nutritional principles." And true to the CIA mission, those principles are used to produce real palate pleasers. How does marinated-grilled chicken breast with spicy apple chutney, whole-wheat spaetzle and mustard jus sound? Or tea-cured pork loin with sweet onion jam and dried morello cherry sauce? These are just two tasty examples of healthy menu items featured at St. Andrew's Café.

Executive chef Rick Moonen, of RM, a seafood restaurant in midtown Manhattan, knows how to write a menu with appetite appeal. He has learned that diners can be scared off by certain words on the menu. So, "crispy" is in. "Deep-fried" is out. The word "cream" has also mysteriously vanished from many restaurant menus, but that doesn't mean it's gone from the kitchen. One more heads-up from Rick Moonen: Poached isn't always the key word for light. His menu offers Butter-Poached Lobster cooked in tons of butter and halibut poached in olive oil. "May I suggest the Grilled Loup de Mer accented with dots of this amazing bright green Greek olive oil?" And, Moonen adds, "If you ask for that fish without any olive oil, you've missed the boat!"

Making Sense of Sauces

While lightening up, chefs have rediscovered the flavor power of broths and infusions. "We poach a steak at Tabla with a black pepper broth, which is delicious," says restaurant owner Danny Meyer. In Houston, the land of the chicken-fried steak, Café Annie offers a culinary oasis where chef/owner Robert Del Grande produces an oven-roasted halibut with hoja santa broth served with sautéed fava beans. "The hoja santa leaves perfume the broth with the fragrance of anise." His advice: "Don't forget to use your spoon." At Bacchanalia and Floataway Café in Atlanta, chef Anne Quatrano laments, "People are frightened by butter and cream. And nobody wants mayonnaise." Their menus do say "a touch of cream" when it's used. A dollop of "aioli" is menu-speak for mayo. But, she says, cooking styles have changed . . . for the better." Instead of heavy butter sauces, dishes feature broths swirled with a small amount of butter, called a "nage."

✳ Restaurant R-E-S-P-E-C-T

Chefs do care about their customers and are willing to make special concessions for special diets, but don't push it. Or no one will be happy with the meal. Café Annie's Robert Del Grande says some diners send him a long list of ingredients to avoid. "Their tickets read like a novel. It's not a prescription; it's a dish I'm cooking." RM's Rick Moonen pleads for sympathy: "Some customers will request no butter, no oil, no carbs, no garlic, no salt, and they add, "Oh and be creative! I want it to taste good!" As long as it's not a life-threatening allergy we're talking about, sometimes it's better to just eat a little less of a chef's specialties if you're concerned about too many high-fat ingredients—rather than trying to reinvent the meal.

FYI: Heavy cream = 45 calories per tablespoon; mayo or butter = 100 calories per tablespoon. Looks like a little cream is the better calorie bargain.

The moral to our menu story? When ordering, don't be afraid to ask what potentially high-fat ingredients might be lurking in your entrée. While words like "broth," "coulis," and "au jus" are green lights for lighter eating, navigating menus isn't always a cinch, because some easy-to-read road signs have been removed.

✳ Hip & Healthy Heroine: Joanne Lichten

Dr. Jo's Restaurant Rules

"It's better to waste it, than to waist it!"—smart advice from fellow foodie and registered dietitian Joanne Lichten, Ph.D., R.D., author of *Dining Lean: How to Eat Out in Your Favorite Restaurants* (Nutrifit, 2000). Joanne, who travels about a hundred days a year, knows how to fit restaurant dining into her on-the-go lifestyle. Her top-two restaurant rules? Rule #1: Beware a False Bargain—don't feel you have to eat the whole thing just because you paid for it. Eating too much will cost you more in terms of extra pounds and bad health down the road. Rule #2: It's Your Dinner—Be Assertive! If you order a dish without butter and it arrives glistening with grease, send it back. If you ordered a sexy red dress from a catalog and they sent you the hideous drab green, wouldn't you return it? Ordering food should be no different.

Oh, Waiter!

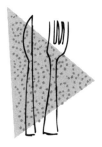

Tips from Tableside Pros on Getting What You Want

1 Listen carefully when they list the specials or tell you about the menu. But it's okay to ask for a replay, if the waiter was on fast-forward.

2 Be specific about what you want or don't want: i.e., "May I have extra lemons for my fish?" "Can you lightly brush the fish with butter?"

3 Remember where you are. Ask for balsamic vinegar in an Italian place and rice wine vinegar in a Japanese place.

4 Be honest when the waiter asks you how you like your meal. Don't suffer in silence. They want to work fast to make you happy.

5 Servings way too large? It's okay to let your server know ahead of time you'll be needing a doggie bag.

6 Make eye contact, smile, and appreciate your server. It's just human nature—waiters are likely to spend more time at friendly tables.

7 Got the absentminded waiter? Okay, not everyone is destined for the hospitality hall of fame. Politely tell the manager what you need.

8 Everybody tip now. It's an industry standard—20 percent for good service.

9 Try to avoid asking for separate checks. Come on now, you can do the math. If not, one of you must have a calculator function on a cell phone or Palm Pilot.

10 Don't forget to say "thanks" to your server. And be sure to tell the manager about the great service, especially if you plan on becoming a regular.

The Healthy Roots of Haute Cuisine

Fancy and fit can live happily ever after. Georges-Auguste Escoffier (1847–1935), the renowned French chef and teacher, was "Da Man!" for haute cuisine. He literally helped launch the modern world of fine dining. But nutrition know-it-alls take note: His philosophy was to mix it up! Keep it interesting! He placed a premium on taste, dishing out perfectly planned courses that provided a parade of flavors and textures. Escoffier would never have dreamed of starting a meal with a cream soup, followed by a fish with beurre blanc sauce and then Bavarian cream for dessert. Following the rules of haute cuisine means creating a balance of light dishes with others that are more sinfully rich. Haute cuisine menus actually embrace healthy choices.

So, you should watch out for the too-much-of-a-good-thing fat trap. It's boring and bulge-producing. Cheese is delicious and adds great flavors to foods, but you don't want to order the Salad with Goat Cheese Croutons, the Seafood Gratin, the broccoli with cheese sauce, and then the cheesecake. Pick one course that says "cheese" (2 tablespoons of shredded Cheddar cheese = about 60 calories).

The same goes for nuts. They are rich in healthy nutrients and heart healthy fats but too much of a good thing is well . . . you know! So, you don't want to order the Almond Citrus Salad, the Macadamia Nut Encrusted Fish, and then the Pecan Pie. Go nutty with one course (1 ounce of nuts = 160 to 200 calories). There's a reason the word *variety* is part of our nutrition mantra, which also includes moderation and balance.

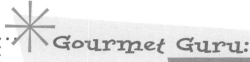

Gourmet Guru:
Chef Charlie Trotter

Flavor Fanatic

Modern-day culinary icon Chef Charlie Trotter, of Charlie Trotter's in Chicago, is famous for his own beautifully orchestrated multicourse meals. **Carolyn Says:** Having dinner at Charlie Trotter's is the evening's entertainment. It's definitely dinner and a show as the courses arrive one by one. Some are the size of two postage stamps and you wonder if he took portion control concerns too seriously! Then you taste and the flavors unfold. Pan-seared Tasmanian salmon with Japanese eggplant, spring peas, and a pea sauce. Or olive oil–poached swordfish with oven-dried tomatoes, roasted white eggplant, and black olives. The descriptions can take longer to say than the dish takes to eat! But with so much care and so many ingredients going into each dish, it inspires the diner to slow down and savor. Then it's on to the next creation. This is what I call a "Temple of Taste."

Charlie puts it this way: "If one pursues flavor first and foremost and works with extraordinarily fresh seasonal foodstuffs, then one is surely going to eat healthy. I prefer to get my good health as a by-product of eating wonderful, tasty, sensual foods that nourish the soul and spirit as well as the body." What's Charlie's favorite food? Vegetables. While others exalt the lobster or caviar on their menus (and Charlie's got plenty of the best on his!) he prefers to look at menu planning the other way. He thinks of the vegetables first. "Vegetables are more interesting, more varied in flavor and texture. They give a dish its character."

Trotter's Tips: Timing is everything! It can never be said too many times, don't overcook vegetables. For example, he says that sliced zucchini, sautéed quickly, should retain a bit of crunch, then add a sprinkling of minced garlic and a splash of vinegar at the very end of cooking. Charlie reveals, "I'm a last-minute fanatic."

Suggested reading: Charlie Trotter's Vegetables (Ten Speed Press, 1996).
Also: *Charlie Trotter's Desserts* (Ten Speed Press, 1998). Happily, Charlie also believes that "Without dessert, it's not a meal!"

What'll It be Tonight?
Chinese, Mexican, Italian?

TIPS FOR HANDLING THE BIG THREE Chinese, Mexican, and Italian are the three most popular ethnic restaurant cuisines. There is a terrific trend nationwide to create more authentic ethnic dishes and often these are much lighter and healthier than the more common souped-up and weighted-down Americanized versions. Our compliments to the chefs who are reintroducing these big flavors that just happen to be healthier. A delicious case in point: Many Chinese restaurants are adding Lettuce Wraps to their menus. A great choice for the crunch, the munch, and the rich Asian flavors of the chicken or shrimp tucked inside.

Chinese

* Start off with wonton, hot and sour, or egg drop soup to curb your appetite.

* Enjoy the green tea! It's calming, fragrant, and research links it to weight control.

* Use chopsticks! It'll slow you down. If you've yet to master the skill, it's high time you did.

* Ask that your dish be stir-fried, using less oil. Each dish is usually made to order.

* Share entrées. In a group, order one less than the number of people. (For the mathematically challenged among us, that comes out to three entrées for four people.)

* Have a little duck sauce, plum sauce, or hoisin to pack more flavor punch. Think of them as Chinese jams and jellies. They are low or no-fat.

* Forgo fried rice or fried noodles. Choose steamed rice or boiled noodles.

* Read your fortune cookie for dessert. Confucius say: "It will add only thirty calories to your meal." (One recently noted exception: Tao, an Asian fusion restaurant in New York City, serves a giant fortune cookie, stuffed with mousse! Calorie count: unknown.)

Eat Less

Fried egg rolls—if an order contains two, eat only one

Sweet and sour entrées—typically battered and deep-fat fried

Cantonese barbecued spareribs—share a few as an appetizer

Crispy beef or Mongolian beef—fried beef

Lemon chicken—battered and deep-fat fried, and topped with syrupy lemon sauce

Kung pao chicken—fried too, one of the highest in fat and calories

Twice-cooked pork—why take another dip in the oil?

Eat More

Steamed dumplings—instead of the fried egg rolls

Steamed Chinese vegetables—if you want them stir-fried, request "a little oil"

Moo goo gai pan—one of the lowest in fat and calories

Chicken or shrimp with snow peas and water chestnuts—lots of veggies is a good thing, bring on the bok choy too!

Hunan (spicy) entrées—usually includes lots of vegetables—again, practice saying: "Use a little oil"

Funky, Fabulous Food Facts

Mmmm, Mmmm, Soup!

Why does soup keep showing up on our menus? Because sipping on soup before you get down to business with the main course makes you eat less. French researchers (what better place to test the theory?) found that soup eaten before lunch, especially if it contained chunks of vegetables, dampened appetite so that people ate fewer calories. They found it worked for both the svelte and zaftig in the study, but for those who fell into the zaftig category, the effects on appetite lingered until dinnertime.

Mexican

* Start off with gazpacho or black bean soup (watch the sour cream garnish).

* Watch out for mindless tortilla chip munching! The basket is there—but beware! Count out a few chips to enjoy with the salsa, which has little or no fat.

* Flavor friends include salsa, picante sauce, pico de gallo, and salsa verde—all made with little or no fat.

* Ask that cheese and sour cream be left off or served on the side and add a touch for flavor.

* Top everything with a healthy helping of shredded lettuce, chopped tomatoes, and pour on the salsa (red or green).

* Tortilla tip: Corn tortillas contain forty less calories than flour tortillas.

* Choose pinto beans or black beans instead of refried beans (they usually have lard thrown in for flavor).

Eat Less

Chicken quesadilla—best shared as an appetizer, go easy on sour cream topping

Chiles rellenos—stuffed, battered, and fried chile peppers

Chimichanga—a fried flour tortilla stuffed with beef, chicken, beans, or cheese

Con queso dip—So tasty! But adds fifty calories with every tablespoon-sized dip in the bowl

Flauta—beef- or chicken-filled fried tortillas, often covered with creamy sauce

Fried ice cream—a relative newcomer to Mexican fare, no explanation needed

Nachos supreme—kind of like biggiesizing; lots o' fat and calories

Refried beans—½ cup contains 250 calories

Sopapillas—fried dough sprinkled with cinnamon and sugar

Taco salad—sure there's some lettuce in there, but mostly meat, cheese, sour cream, and guacamole in a fried tortilla shaped like a bowl (Ole!— the bowl alone adds over 400 calories!)

Eat More

Arroz con pollo—chicken with rice

Chicken enchiladas—corn tortillas filled with chicken and served with tomato-based sauce

Fajitas—grilled beef, chicken, or shrimp with peppers and onions; you control how much cheese or sour cream to put on each tortilla

Fish tacos—popularized in Southern California, often served with tasty slaw

Grilled fish—many Mexican restaurants feature great grilled fish with fresh lime and spicy salsas

Mexican rice—flavorful side dish—½ cup contains 150 calories

Soft tacos—grilled beef or chicken wrapped in flour tortilla

The United Tastes of America

One of the most wonderful things about the U.S.A. is the melting pot of cultures and cuisines. It's a taste adventure to join friends in your own hometown for a meal starring the foods of Morocco, Thailand, Greece, Vietnam, Sweden, Argentina, or any number of deliciously different world cuisines. Rather than giving you a whole list of the do's and don'ts for each and every mouthwatering cuisine, what's in order here is sharing a basic food adventure philosophy. If you don't know what something is, ASK. If you've never had it before, TRY IT. If you don't like it, TRY SOMETHING ELSE. Some cuisines feature more grilled items and some more fried. Some lay on the cream, others never touch the stuff. So, it really pays to study the menu ahead of time. And if you're going with a friend who happens to be from this faraway place—they're the best gourmet guides.

Italian

∗ Start off with minestrone soup. An Italian vegetable soup classic!

∗ Avoid pastas stuffed with cheese. Enjoy the flavor of freshly grated Parmesan cheese sprinkled on top.

∗ Be sauce savvy. Alfredo sauce is made with butter, heavy cream, and Parmesan cheese.

∗ Yes! Olive oil is heart healthy. But avoid an oil spill. It's still all fat, so it adds significant calories.

∗ Pass on Eggplant Parmigiana—battered, fried, and topped with cheese.

∗ Balsamic vinegar is terrific! This aged vinegar adds *molto gusto* (a whole lot 'a flavor!) to salads.

∗ Italians love flavor, by the way. Take advantage of that culinary culture and seek out dishes with rosemary, basil, red peppers, artichokes, capers, and lemon.

Eat Less

Butter sauces—lemon butter, marsala wine butter, pesto butter

Cheese manicotti—lots of cheese; if you must have it, share with friends

Fettucine alfredo—In Italy, they would share a plate of this among six people

Fried calamari—share as appetizer and enjoy with lemon and marinara sauce

Lasagna—It's filling for a reason!

Light tomato sauce—See the light! It actually means prepared with cream to make it a lighter color

Parmigiana—chicken, veal, or eggplant—it's battered, fried, and topped with cheese

Eat More

Chicken cacciatore—tomato-based sauce with onion, wine, and fresh herbs

Fish florentine—means served with spinach

Pasta with marinara or pomodoro sauces—tomato-based

Puttanesca—dishes prepared with tomato, capers, and anchovies

Primavera—means springtime in Italian, lots of vegetables

Red clam sauce—less calories and fat than white clam sauce

Flaunt Your Good Taste—for Food or Fashion

High-fat, high-flavor ingredients such as olive oil, butter, cheeses, cream, bacon, nuts, and fried foods are ooh-la-la delicious . . . but treat them as you would flashy fashion accessories. Be choosy. Just the right necklace or belt accents your look. Too many baubles and bangles weigh you down. Apply the fashion philosophy of the late, great French fashion icon, Coco Chanel, to meals: "Get dressed" (serve your plate) "and then remove at least one accessory" (one side dish, dessert, or bread). "Then you'll be just right."

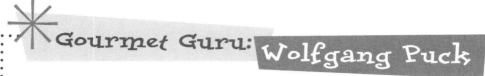

Gourmet Guru: Wolfgang Puck

Glitz and Glamour Meet Good Health

Carolyn Says: Wolfgang Puck's cooking style and spirit of taste adventure helped revitalize, reinvent, and add flavor pizzaz to American restaurant food. (Even if it did arrive with an Austrian accent!) I am not sure what impressed me the most about my first visit to Spago, Hollywood. Was it the bright, welcoming personality of the charming and creative chef, Wolfgang Puck? "Hey! Miss CNN, how about a smoked salmon and caviar pizza?"

Or, was it the way the Sunset Boulevard–view dining room, dotted with flashy celebs, was ironically outfitted with casual white patio furniture? "Isn't that Milton Berle waiting at the hostess stand? Is that Mickey Rourke sitting next to us? I think that's Michael Eisner over there. And Tony Curtis at the bar?" This was Hollywood!

Okay, I confess. It was the food! Never had I tasted tomatoes with so much flavor dressed with a sprinkling of crunchy sea salt, aged balsamic vinegar, and fragrant extra-virgin olive oil. Arugula and radicchio salad! Free-range chicken with Chardonnay and fresh herbs! Angel hair pasta tossed with goat cheese and sun-dried tomatoes! Ingredients we take for granted today, and can add to our shopping carts almost anywhere, were just beginning to pop and sizzle. Wolfgang Puck, on the curl of this culinary wave, opened his kitchen so diners could see him perform and paint their plates with the bright colors of red pepper coulis and jewel green basil oil. Salads became a celebration of California's bounty, introducing the handcrafted beauty of organic produce. Golden beets! Who knew?

Desserts were elevated beyond gooey sugar and fat to become stars in their own right, pairing the real flavors of peach and apple and plums with the crunch of perfect pastry. Long live the menus of Spago!—even more creative today as Wolfgang Puck's culinary influence shepherds a new generation of chefs twirling pizzas and tossing salads at his many restaurants. Spago, Beverly Hills is Puck's epicenter of success today with award-winning executive chef Lee Hefter at the helm. But I still kinda miss the lawn chairs.

American Beauties—
Tips to Keep You in That Category Too!

✳ *Fast Food Lane*—It can be green light, go! But don't turn off the caution lights completely. Fast-food places dotted along the nation's highways and on every corner of every town offer standardization and convenience. And we're not just talking about the rest rooms! A growing number offer salads, grilled chicken, veggie burgers, and reasonably sized basic burgers. Skip the bacon, extra cheese, and goopy sauces and ask for extra lettuce, tomato, pickles, and onions, if that's your pleasure. You've heard it before—but it bears repeating—beware biggiesizing, supersizing, and supervalue combo meals, or your body might be supersized too! Gotta have fries? Memorize this line: "and I'll have a *small* order of fries, please." To add a serving of fruit, choose a container of orange juice, available now anytime of day.

✳ Put fast food on the menu more than twice a week and you may boost your odds of not just putting on a few extra pounds, but achieving the big "O"—Obesity!

Based on Research by Mark Pereira, Ph.D., Harvard Medical School

✳ *Family Fast Casual*—This is the fastest-growing category in the restaurant industry. TGI Friday's is credited with making it a nationwide phenom, but now large-chain restaurants offering moderately priced menus, consistent quality, friendly service, and a festive atmosphere are taking the lead in responding to customers' demands for healthier dishes in a big way. For instance, Olive Garden has added Healthy Fare menu items, which are lower in fat and calories. You can even find the nutrition profile of these dishes on the restaurant's website: *www.olivegarden.com.* Because these restaurants are used to big tables of families and friends, servers are usually used to requests to share appetizers, split entrées, and fetch boxes for leftovers. But these are also the eateries known for value and that often means huge portions at easy-to-swallow prices. The Cheesecake Factory is infamous for its mega servings. Even the Caesar salad is made with multiple heads of romaine lettuce! So, enjoy, but be prepared to ask servers to describe portion sizes so you can work out what to order and what to split with your dining buddies. Many of these restaurants have open kitchens now so you might even wander by the cooks in action to actually check out portion sizes before you order.

✳ *Sandwich Shops*—How about a nice sandwich for lunch? Sounds innocent enough, but when it arrives with the ham and cheese about three inches thick and a huge scoop of potato salad on the side—it's not the bread you should be worried about! You should shoot for no more than three ounces of meat on your sandwich. Each one-ounce slice of cheese adds an additional 100 calories. Build sandwich bulk with lettuce, tomatoes, and sprouts, and add flavor with mustards—which are basically calorie-free—or vinegar-and-oil-based dressings. And you're not the only one looking for a great-tasting healthy sandwich. Nationwide chains, most notably Subway, have created new sub sandwiches especially designed to maximize flavor and minimize fat. Go to *www.subway.com* and see for yourself how many subs have less than 6 grams of fat, including the Sweet Onion Chicken Teriyaki and the Red Wine Vinaigrette Club. But, *ahoy, matey!*—there's something big on the line—the six-inch classic tuna sub weighs in at 22 grams of fat. Again, you've gotta know the facts, before you choose your food.

Hold *the* Mayo?

Sorry we couldn't give you the nutritional analysis of all the sandwich combinations out there. (That would be a book by itself.) According to calculations done by the National Restaurant Association, a sandwich consisting of just five possible items or toppings, i.e., bread, meat, cheese, lettuce, and tomato, can be ordered 120 ways. A sandwich comprised of ten possible items could come in 3,628,800 combinations. Want more options? A sandwich that offers fifteen possible items has 1.3 trillion combinations. So, in the restaurant world not all nutrition labeling is possible. But that doesn't mean eateries shouldn't give Nutrition 101 the old college try! Most chain restaurants have very specific recipes for their regular menu items, so it sure would be helpful if they provided the nutrition breakdown, if not on the menu, on a brochure or at least on their websites. Au Bon Pain is even starting to put nutrition information on self-service computer kiosks in some of their stores so you see what you're eating. You may not always like what you see, but sticker shock can help you make diet decisions. Did you know that some fast-food salads (piled high with fried chicken strips, bacon, cheese, and creamy salad dressings) can contain more fat and calories than the regular-size burger and fries? Who knew? Nobody! Until they read the nutrition information!

* *Breakfast Eatery*—yes, breakfast is the healthy way to start the day (see chapter 2, The Dish on Diet Basics, for more), but when "Let's go out for breakfast" turns into a cheese omelet, hash browns, bacon, sausage, and biscuits slathered in butter, you've moved into the budget-busting calorie category. A three-egg ham-and-cheese omelet can rack up five hundred calories (or more) on its own. And you wanted a side of silver-dollar pancakes with that? Instead, order a small veggie omelet with just a sprinkle of Cheddar cheese on top, enjoy a glass of orange juice, a slice of whole-wheat toast thinly spread with butter or your favorite spread, and order the fresh fruit cup or grapefruit half. Yes, they ate big breakfasts back on the farm—but most of us today don't have to plow the north forty before noon.

✳ Croissant Caution

A three-ounce croissant, as dainty and elegant as it may sound, contains the fat equivalent of four pats of butter, before you even start slathering on the mayo. Croissants are in the lip-smacking-good pastry family and are among the most calorie-laden choices you can select for your sandwich. That three-ounce croissant—and many sandwich shops offer much larger ones—racks up 360 calories. Now you know!

✳ *Steak House*—believe it or not, steak restaurants can be among the easiest places to choose a healthy meal. You get to pick a steak that's petite (may we suggest the filet mignon, *sans* the bacon wrapping?), there are usually delicious salads on the menu, and most side dishes are served à la carte so you can choose the steamed broccoli without the cheese sauce and enjoy one half of a baked potato, if you like. Just don't count that huge stack of onion rings as your daily five vegetable servings. Those deep-fat-fried whole onion creations served at some steak places can set you back almost two-thousand calories (à la Bloomin' Onion at Outback). Woah, Pardner! On the plus side, if you're not in the mood for meat, most steak houses offer chicken and pork loin (the leanest cut of pork). Many have a great selection of fresh fish too.

✳ *Seafood Place*—okay, just because you've set sail for seafood doesn't mean all of the menu choices are going to keep you shipshape. Beware the deep-fat-fried, drowned-in-butter, and smothered-in-cream-sauce seafood dishes. Choose broiled, grilled, or baked fish with your new restaurant-ordering skills and ask that "the fish be just brushed with butter or oil." Go easy on the fries and choose the rice pilaf and veggies as side dishes. Steamed or grilled shrimp is a great low-fat choice enjoyed with cocktail sauce, which you can use freely. (It's the tartar sauce and rémoulade sauce, which are mainly mayo.) Now, a seafood quiz:

Guess which is higher in fat: New England Clam Chowder or Manhattan Clam Chowder? You're right—New England, the one with all the cream! Really got to have the New England style? Ask for a cup, not a bowl. Seafood cioppino is a good soup choice too, since it's chock full of fish and veggies in a tomato-based broth.

Gourmet Guru: Eric Ripert

Seafood Savvy

Do you crave the taste of filet mignon served with creamy and rich béarnaise sauce but would rather not pay the cost in calories and cholesterol? Well, Eric Ripert, the brilliant (and male-model handsome) co-owner and executive chef of Le Bernardin restaurant in New York City, created a just-as-delicious alternative fresh from the sea, Seared Tuna Paillard with Tarragon Vinaigrette. A meaty fresh tuna steak is sliced thin (paillard-style), seared on one side, and finished with a drizzle of tarragon vinaigrette. Your taste buds won't miss the beef with béarnaise, but your waistline sure will know the difference. Maguy Le Coze, founder and co-owner of Le Bernardin, is perhaps the best example of how enjoying this lighter style of French cuisine pays off in compliments! The menu earns top marks from restaurant reviewers and helps Maguy remain film star svelte in her elegant French couture. Maguy says, "That's the magic of Eric!" Ripert, who is from the South of France, prepares seafood with a lighter touch using olive oil, garlic, and herbs rather than the heavier cream-based dishes of northern France. "If you cook fish too rich you hide the flavors."

He shares his genius with mere kitchen mortals in his classy cookbook and is passionate about demanding the freshest ingredients. Carolyn Says: While shooting a segment for CNN on seafood I spent the morning in the kitchens of Le Bernardin. Eric opened boxes of live fish flown in overnight from Maine. He showed me scallops so fresh they were still wriggling in their shells and explained, "It's the best to get seafood that is alive. The fish and shellfish will be sweet and taste like the ocean. And the texture will be moist and firm." Maguy! Lunch at Le Bernardin every day? We would love to be in your shoes! Designer stilettos perhaps?

Suggested reading: A Return to Cooking, Eric Ripert (Artisan, 2002).

Rare Seared Tuna Paillard Topped with a Salad of Baby Watercress with Shallot-Tarragon Vinaigrette, String Beans, and Olives

Eric Ripert, chef Le Bernardin restaurant, New York City

YIELD: *6 servings*

The Vinaigrette:

1½ teaspoons minced shallots

3 tablespoons sherry vinegar

1 teaspoon Dijon mustard

½ teaspoon fine sea salt

Pinch of freshly ground white
  pepper

½ cup olive oil

1 tablespoon chopped tarragon

The Tuna:

½ pounds haricots verts, trimmed

30 niçoise olives, pitted and halved

12 red cherry tomatoes, halved

12 yellow cherry tomatoes, halved

Two 8-ounce tuna steaks (about
  1 inch thick)

2 tablespoons extra-virgin olive oil

Fine sea salt and freshly ground
  white pepper to taste

1 tablespoon thyme leaves

2 tablespoons thinly sliced chives

1 lemon, halved and seeded

½ pound baby watercress (or
  mesclun greens)

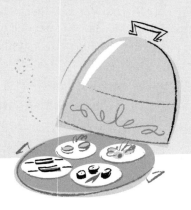

1. For the vinaigrette, whisk together in a small bowl the shallots, vinegar, mustard, salt, and pepper until the salt dissolves. Constantly whisking, slowly drizzle in the olive oil. Store in the refrigerator until ready to use.

2. Bring a pot of water to a boil and salt generously. Blanch the haricots verts until crisp-tender, about 5 minutes. Strain and then run under cold water until chilled. Set aside.

3. For the salad, place the haricots verts, olives, red and yellow tomatoes in a bowl and season with salt and pepper. Add the tarragon to the vinaigrette and whisk to combine. Toss the vegetables with enough vinaigrette to coat and divide evenly around the rim of six plates.

4. For the tuna, cut each steak into three equal slices (about 1 inch thick). Place two nonstick pans over high heat. When the pans are hot, brush the tuna with olive oil on each side. Season generously with the salt and pepper. Sprinkle with the thyme leaves. Add the tuna to the pans and sear on both sides until nicely browned but still rare, about 30 seconds on each side. Remove from the pan.

5. Sprinkle the tuna with the chives. Place a tuna slice in the center of each plate. Squeeze the lemon juice over the tuna. Toss the watercress with enough vinaigrette to coat and season to taste with salt and pepper. Divide the salad evenly and mound on top of the tuna. Serve immediately.

✳ *All You Can Eat Buffet*—*Viva Las Vegas, Baby!* The secret here is to scope out the entire spread before grabbing your plate and piling it high as you move along the line. Try to keep it in perspective. Think of your buffet-style meal as a meal, not a free-for-all. Choose the salad course, the entrée, the vegetables, the starch side dish, and of course save room for dessert. On good buffets (they're actually rated in Vegas!) you should find some steamed shrimp to start and roast beef being carved for each customer. These lean protein choices are a good base for your buffet. And what's great about a buffet is that you can see the foods before choosing. You don't have to depend on a menu description. Of course an eye check is not always enough to identify fat and calorie content. So, try to avoid the steam table pans of things swimming in cream or cheese sauces. Buffets also offer you creative freedom. You can even design your own vegetarian meal, with a dizzying number of veggie side dishes to choose from. Want more than one dessert? Go ahead and sample a bunch! Just don't take a full serving of each. A sliver of cheesecake, a thin, thin slice of key lime pie, one small square of double chocolate cake, a spoonful of raspberry mousse. That's the food freedom of the buffet. You can take what you want, sample more tastes, and maintain control over portion sizes.

Hip & Healthy Heroine: Elizabeth Blau

The Real Vegas Show Girl

Who knew that Las Vegas was a go-to town for great food and fitness? Yes, even in this epicenter of sin, where smoking, drinking, gambling, and staying up all night are the rule, rather than the exception (casinos have no clocks, you know), it's easy to find healthy menu items and places to work out in style. The MGM Grand's state-of-the-art fitness facilities overlook palm tree vistas and acres of swimming pools while high-energy music keeps you motivated on the treadmill. Then it's off to the Spa where a good soak, hot steam, and a massage put you back together again for another night on the town.

Beyond the anything-you-want buffets, Las Vegas has upped the ante on fine dining with a myriad of super restaurants where celebrity chefs get top billing on casino marquees right next to big-name entertainers. "That translates into more choices for health-conscious foodies who crave elegant dining," says Elizabeth Blau, the striking, supermodel tall, food and beverage executive who helped recreate the culinary landscape of Las Vegas. "We lured great restaurateurs, like Sirio Maccioni, to open Vegas versions of Le Cirque and Circo in the Bel Agio Hotel and Casino." Other great chefs followed. Elizabeth now works her menu magic as a partner in Simon's Kitchen and Bar at the Hard Rock Hotel. Carolyn Says: Okay, it was a splurge, but the truffle-scented, perfectly prepared fries at Simon's are over-the-moon fantastic. I shared an order with three gal pals as I dined on a succulent veal chop served with earthy exotic mushrooms. BTW: They also serve the freshest and crunchiest baby spinach and endive salad. Yum! Another Vegas winner, Noodles, in the Bel Agio Hotel, where we savored spicy Thai Shrimp Noodle bowls scented with lemongrass and served with baby bok choy. So can you stay fit on your Vegas vacation? You can bet on it.

10 Slim-and-Trim Restaurant Rules

1 **Be prepared.** Okay, so you're not cooking, but that doesn't mean you shouldn't know what's for dinner. Read the menu ahead of time. You can even check out the menu on some restaurants' websites so you can really plan ahead. Or take time to look it over while you are waiting for the table. (If it's the latest trendy hot spot, you could be there a while!) You spent quality time planning what you were going to wear, why not do the same for what you're going to eat?

2 **Breathe in, breathe out.** If you are famished when you arrive, first take a deep-cleansing breath. Don't be suckered in by Chad's chirpy sales pitch to "start with the spinach cheese dip or chili nachos while you're deciding on your entrée." Instead, order a sparkling water or a nonalcoholic "mocktail" to get the party started. (Check out chapter 6 for The Dish on Drinks.)

3 **Ask, and ye shall receive.** Read the menu and ask the waiter for descriptions of dishes, including how they are prepared. Do they use a lot of butter on the broiled fish? Is the cauliflower soup cream-based? If so, can you get a cup instead of a bowl?

4 **Have an appetizer party.** Lots of dishes means lots of tastes for everyone to share, and chances are you won't eat as much as you would if the whole dish was plopped in front of you. Many restaurants are actually designing their dishes to be shared. The waiter should know this. It's easy to split an order of four Thai Shrimp Spring Rolls, but a tad more challenging to share a bowl of Thai Coconut Chicken Soup.

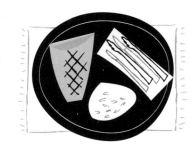

5   **Check out the room.** Look around and see what other diners are eating, so you get a visual on portion sizes. It pays to spy. If portions are huge, you can split the entrée or even ask the waiter to serve you half and box the rest to take home for later. You'll also get to see that the "served with baby spring greens" is either a sizable serving of salad or a disappointing wisp of lettuce meant to be a garnish.

6   **What's the rush?** Put the fork down every once in a while. Savor the flavors. Remember to breathe between bites and actually talk to your dinner mates. A sip of wine between bites enhances dining and digestion as well. Pinpoint the way your Pinot Noir matches so nicely with the duck or lamb. See how the Sauvignon Blanc livens up the grilled seafood.

7   **Don't like your dish? Trade it in.** If your meal is just so-so, or isn't what you thought it was going to be, order something else. Or if you've had your fill—stop eating. This is not the clean-plate club. If the grouper needs something and you don't want to lather on more tartar sauce, ask for lemons or hot sauce if that's your thing. Heck, the balsamic vinaigrette meant for the salad might even be the best request to rescue your fish.

8   **Sauce on the side works . . . sometimes.** Béarnaise sauce at steak restaurants usually comes in a huge gravy boat, best kept *way* on the side. But if the sauce is a light swirl and part of the chef's creative vision, enjoy it the way it's intended to be. You don't have to eat the whole thing.

The Dish

9 **Healthy color is key.** Think of your plate as a color palette. The more color—the better. That's code for: Eat your fruits and vegetables! Yes, sometimes it's what you add to a meal that makes it healthy, not what you avoid. Many restaurants today have incredible seasonally fresh vegetable side dishes and salads. Why not ask for these to be biggiesized? If they freely offer huge portions of French fries, why not a double portion of steamed broccoli or green beans? Go easy on cream-sauced, cheese-slathered, buttery-rich, and deep-fat fried versions.

10 **Check, please.** Always be sure to top off a really good meal with, "My compliments to the chef!" for menu additions you loved and thank anyone else who made your special requests a reality. Even if you're not a regular, maybe you're just visiting the town, let the restaurant staff know you appreciate their terrific service. And even if your journeys never take you to Jackson Hole or Jacksonville again, your constructive culinary comments might help the next gal on the road. We can see it now, a nation united by "sauce on the side!"

✳ Dinner *and* a movie? Dinner was fabulous. Now you're ready to take in a movie. Better check out chapter 10 first.—Carolyn and Densie

Was It Something You Ate?
When Good Food Goes Bad.

You had what seemed like a great meal, but you think you've followed it up with a twenty-four-hour virus or a touch of the flu. Think again. Chances are it might have been bad bugs in something you ate. While restaurant employees are often trained in food safety and sanitation (ask if the restaurant participates in the National Restaurant Association's Serve Safe Program), you should keep an eye out for signs of potential trouble. Salmonella bacteria is the most common culprit, but there are many other potential pathogens in mishandled foods. And this isn't a rare occurrence, with an estimated 76 million cases of food-borne illness each year. Anyone who's been there can tell you, it's no fun. In fact, it's potentially life threatening. Experts recommend you call the doctor. Don't try to tough it out on your own. Medical care givers can help you feel better sooner.

Five Signs a Restaurant Is Serving Safe Foods

1 Dining room is clean. What you see is what you get. (If tables, chairs, utensils, and glasses aren't clean, chances are things aren't too clean in the kitchen either.)

2 Restrooms are clean. This is an important indicator. Attention to detail is a very good thing.

3 Staff dressed neat and clean. Beware the food handler who also handles the cash. Those greenbacks are a breeding ground for all kinds of yucky stuff.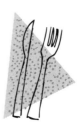

4 Health inspection certificate displayed. If they don't make the grade, make tracks!

5 Cold food is cold and the hot food is hot. Lukewarm foods lurk in the danger zone, where bacteria love to grow—40 degrees to 140 degrees F.

Doggie Bags: Taking Care of Your Carryout

Okay, so it's not really for your dog. Wrapping up leftovers is a great way to limit portion sizes and have a great little lunch the next day. But take care of that food on your way home.

✳ Insist on a specially designed takeout container. Most restaurants are using sturdy, easy-to-seal plastic or Styrofoam containers. No flimsy bags, please.

✳ Foods should not be left unrefrigerated for more than two hours, one hour if it's more than 90 degrees outside.

✳ Reheat leftovers to 165 degrees until hot and steaming.

✳ Don't have a clue what the temperature is or how long you've had it in the fridge? When in doubt, throw it out! Trust us on this one. You're better off safe than sick.

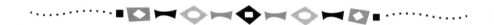

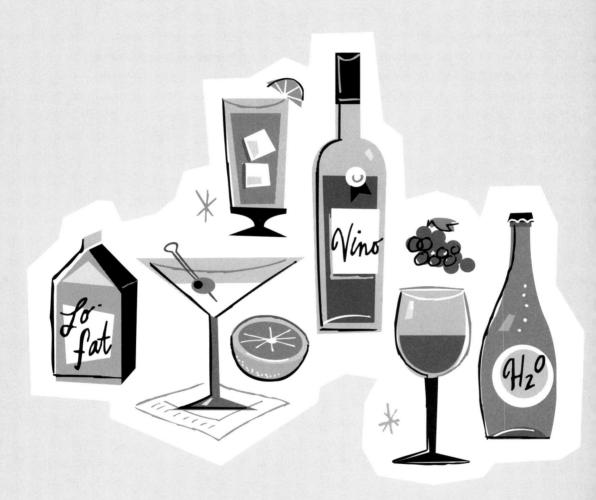

6 The Dish on Drinks

Drinks—*the one culinary category* that's often overlooked in dietary do's and don'ts. It's way too easy to convince yourself that the calories you quaff just don't count. But count they do. On the flip side, beverages can be terrific sources of healthy nutrients. Think milk, juice, and fruit smoothies. And, yes, a glass of wine with dinner can be good for your heart. You just have to know which drinks in what amounts are going to dish up that healthy inner glow you seek. So, here we take on the liquid portion of portion control! From sports drinks to water, milk to Merlot, let's pour over some beverage basics. Hey, our philosophy works here too. The more you know, the more you can drink and the more choices you have to satisfy your thirst, or imbibe without overdoing! Digest this liquid logic: Did you know that one cup of eggnog contains *more than twice* the number of calories in a glass of Chardonnay (not to mention the fact that it carries a hefty load of saturated fats, while Chardonnay is fat-free)? So, shy away from a mug

> These pretzels are making me thirsty.
> —Jerry Seinfeld

of that holiday eggnog—unless you're ready to stop the party there. (We prefer the calorie-free eggnog option offered at the decidedly upscale Paul Labrecque Spa in New York for $115—an eggnog bath, complete with cinnamon and nutmeg slathered all over your body! We kid you not.) Okay, so a sip or two is okay, if your holiday isn't complete without it. The same holds true for any drink. An occasional soda, a fruit smoothie, a gin and tonic. Nothing is off limits; you just gotta know what you're downing. The bottom line: Beverages you choose (and how much you drink) can make or break a healthy diet. So read on and drink up.

Water

While we've already introduced you to the wonderful world of water in chapter 2, now we're taking it to the next level. It's a supply-and-demand thing. Companies are supplying more and more bottled water choices and women are demanding to know which ones are best. It's no walk in the waterpark, out there. You have your vitamin-fortified waters, herb-enhanced waters, tea-infused waters, soy waters, bacteria-enhanced waters (like the good bacteria you find in yogurt), caffeine-laced waters, fiber-enriched waters, flavored waters, and last, but not least, if you can even believe it, artificially sweetened waters—the best we can make of this concoction is it's a diet drink in disguise. The price for such fanciful H_2Os, sometimes gently referred to as "enhanced" waters, can run you as much as $2.00 a bottle. But price isn't even the point. If you're looking to boost your water intake, do you really need all these bells and whistles being offered as part of the package? We think not.

Having Your Way with Water: Check the Nutrition Facts label. Does it provide any calories? If it does, then it's not water; it's a sweetened drink. Water should be calorie-free, period. Sweetened waters can add an extra fifty calories for an eight-ounce glass. And if it's artificially sweetened, ask yourself—what's the difference between an artificially sweetened bottle of water and an artificially sweetened can of soda—a few bubbles, perhaps? Skip it.

Next: If it's fortified with vitamins and minerals, you might want to rethink your purchase. Is this really necessary? If you're following our guidelines to eat healthy foods (feel free to refresh your memory by backtracking to chapter 2) and you're taking a multi, plus a calcium supplement, it's really tough to justify spending the extra cash on fortified waters. They're not a bad thing, just not a necessary part of your newly pumped up healthy diet. Most provide anywhere from 10 to 100 percent of your daily recommended intake for the nutrients they contain. But they contain only a handful of nutrients—nowhere near as many individual vitamins and minerals as you'd get from a multi, or even a serving of fortified cereal.

Choosing a bottled water is really more a matter of taste than nutrition. There are some subtle taste differences, but you'll have to do your own personal taste test to find a winner. Looking for "pure spring water" or something equally wholesome-sounding? Good luck. You can't always depend on labels to give you a clear picture of what the source of the water really is. Lots of bottled water labels boast that they're pure, natural, pristine, clean, come from mountain water, or are naturally occurring. But it's a crap shoot as to whether they really are what they claim. While some do come from natural springs (picture Rocky Mountain high, here), it's certainly not the rule. That "pure" water you're paying a premium for could also have come from a municipal water supply—25 percent of bottled water actually does—and been rebottled with an attractive label rather than the more honest "this water comes from a municipal water supply and has been rebottled to make it more appealing."

Whichever form of water you choose, just remember our 8 x 8 recommendation (eight 8-ounce glasses of water a day).

Soft Drinks

. . . .

While diet soft drinks may be popular because they offer zero calories, they offer zero nutrition, too. A daily diet drink is probably okay, but think of it as a filler, not a food. Most of our experts insist artificial sweeteners are safe, but the truth is, no one really knows for sure. Our take on it? Artificial sweeteners, like aspartame (NutraSweet), saccharin (Sweet 'N Low), and sucralose (Splenda) in small amounts (one or two diet drinks a day) is probably safe for almost everyone. But who knows if some people might suffer health problems down the road from drinking five, six, or seven cans of the stuff a day. Maybe you haven't noticed, but when you're trying to skimp on food, it's easy to down several cans of your diet drink *du jour*. If diet drinks will never pass your lips and you prefer the taste of regular cola, ginger ale, or other soft drinks, add them to your day as you would a candy treat or a dessert splurge. (For more info on artificial sweeteners, check out chapter 4, The Dish on Eating In.)

✳ Sweet Nothings on the Label

Densie Says: If you're a voracious label reader like me, you may have noticed that diet drinks sweetened with saccharin no longer carry labels proclaiming that the sweetener may be "hazardous to your health." Does that mean that saccharin has been given a squeaky clean bill of health? Not exactly. Turns out that, in its infinite wisdom, Congress decided (Who knew? No one asked us) to allow products containing the artificial sweetener to go warning-free, and it's no longer considered an official "suspected carcinogen." Here's the dish: Some experts still think there's reason for concern and caution against using saccharin at all. It's just a little more difficult to spot as an ingredient now. The only way to know now is to check out the mice type on the back of the label to see if saccharin is in any of the products you're buying.

Juice

Fruit juice is good for you, right? Well, the answer is yes, *if* what you're sipping is 100 percent fruit juice. But there are so many fruit-juice wannabes out there vying for your attention, it's hard for even us to keep track. When you opt for 100 percent fruit juice, like orange juice, grapefruit juice, pear juice, tomato juice, prune juice, or a vegetable blend, like V8, you're getting the most nutrition bang for your buck. Anything else offers less stellar nutrition numbers and a cleverly disguised dose of sugar. Citrus juices are especially good sources of vitamins and phytonutrients and, if they're calcium-fortified, a great way to get your calcium. In fact, the kind of calcium added to some orange juices, Tropicana for instance, is called Citrical and is very easily absorbed by the body, so it can really help build and keep strong bones. The only downside to fruit juice? You don't get the fiber fix you get from whole fruits. So be sure to mix it up. Some juice, some whole fruit, and you'll be fine. Just so you'll know, six ounces of fruit juice is considered a serving.

Pulp Fiction

Be choosey. Go for 100 percent juices only. The terms "beverage," "cocktail," "drink," and "punch" are dead giveaways that it's not 100 percent juice. While "juice" may be splashed across the label, if it doesn't say 100 percent juice, it could contain as little as 5 to 10 percent of the real deal. The rest is probably water and high-fructose corn syrup. Not the supernutrition you were hoping for!

Lowest calorie fruit juice: tomato—clocks in at only about thirty calories in a six-ounce glass. But it is also the highest in sodium—something to keep top of mind if you're trying to keep bloating to a minimum. Next lowest? Grapefruit juice at seventy-five calories in a six-ounce glass.

✳ **Carolyn Says:** **Grapefruit juice is my personal favorite, because it's so refreshing. And not only is it one of the lowest-calorie juices, filled with hundreds of healthy nutrients, studies have shown that it acts as a natural diuretic to reduce bloating. Talk about a girl's best friend!**

Highest-calorie fruit juice: prune—racks up about 135 calories per six-ounce glass, but don't write it off. It's one of the most antioxidant-packed foods around and works natural wonders to keep you regular.

To Juice or Not to Juice

What about juicing it yourself? There are two sides to the juicing coin. On the plus side is taste. Nothing can compare with the flavor of a freshly prepared glass of juice either squeezed (orange) or juiced (carrot). The downside to the do-it-yourself approach is the time it takes to prepare all that fresh-from-the-fruit taste. It's your call. If you have the time, by all means go for fresh. But don't feel like you're getting inferior nutrition by grabbing the stuff in a carton. Either way will get you great nutrition; which path you choose to get there is up to you. *Food Safety Note:* Unlike most packaged juices, fresh-squeezed juices are not pasteurized to kill potential bacteria that might be clinging to the fruit you throttle through the juicer, so drink them soon after preparation and always refrigerate any extra juice promptly.

True Food Confessions

Juice It Up

Densie Says: I love fresh carrot juice. I'd drink it every day—if someone else would prepare it for me! All that peeling and juicing. It takes a pound or two of carrots to get a decent-size glass. And then there's the cleanup. All that orange gunk to be wiped out and tossed. Don't get me started. Okay, here's the confession part. I have a $200+ juicer that has been retired to the back of a bottom cabinet in my kitchen, for the simple reason that fresh juice just takes too much time to prepare. I plan to bring it out of retirement soon. Maybe as soon as we finish this book. But take my advice. Make sure you're ready, willing, and able to devote the time it takes to be a serious juicer chick before you fork over a wad of your hard-earned dough for such a task-specific kitchen appliance.

Coffee

. . . .

Java, cuppa joe, café. Whatever you call it, a couple of decades has made a big difference. (For better or worse, the godfather of all coffee chains, Starbucks, was launched in 1985.) Today, your coffee choice is more than just a coffee break; it makes a statement about who you are. Are you a latte lady, a cappuccino chick, or a mocha madam? But while your choice of café may convey something about your character, these days, it can also define your waistline. A calorie-free cup of java has morphed into something that more resembles a triple-malted than a cup of coffee. These bloated coffee drinks have been dubbed "food porn" by some nutritionist activists. It's tough to argue with that label. Since when is a cup of coffee supposed to weigh twenty ounces and provide a calorie count on the other side of eight hundred? Basically, you're ordering a big fat dessert, not taking a coffee break. Think about it. Opt instead for your more subtly flavored coffee choices—café latte, café Americano, vanilla latte—and ask for skim milk. If fat-free milk just doesn't cut it with your taste buds, then go for whole milk and ask for a small cuppa. Or if you really want to get down to basics, just put blinders on to all those whipped cream, chocolate, mocha, caramel, and toffee-topped drinks and order the coffee of the day.

✳ For Politically Correct Coffee Drinkers

No, it's not an unintentional oxymoron. You can drink your coffee and still keep your PC environmental conscience clear. We have two words for you: shade-grown coffee. Coffee plants actually grow naturally in the protective shade of tropical and subtropical forests around the world. But the plants grow faster and produce more coffee beans in the sun. To let in the light (and boost the bottom line), coffee growers are knocking down trees, which of course, affects the natural forest wildlife. So there you have it. Buy coffee grown in the shade and you may have saved trees and wildlife, especially birds. That explains why one major mail-order brand of shade-grown coffee has been dubbed Song Bird Coffee. You can find shade-grown coffee at some Whole Foods, Safeway, Albertson's, Thriftway, or Trader Joe's, as well as coffee houses (yes, Starbucks carries it), or online.

Coffee Weighs In

Coffee has somewhat of a schizophrenic reputation when it comes to dieting. While in some coffee klatches it's thought of as a diet aid, of sorts, kicking your metabolism up a notch to burn fat and calories at a faster clip, it's also been banished to the "do-not-eat" list by some celebrity diet book authors (whose names we shall not mention), who say it's a toxic substance that's bad for your body and a creator of cravings. The truth lies somewhere in between. No one would argue the fact that coffee contains caffeine, a stimulant. And stimulants do rev up the metabolism. In fact, a jolt of caffeine is a common ingredient in over-the-counter weight-loss supplements, along with any number of herbs. But the caffeine in a cup of coffee or in a weight-loss supplement is not enough to make much of a difference in your weight; neither is it likely to send sugar cravings into orbit.

Coffee Cons

Coffee has been the subject of an intense investigation over the last few decades that would put to shame any done by the CIA, the KGB, or the Israeli Mossad. But still, no smoking gun, much to the consternation of coffee haters everywhere. Here's the dish on coffee and your health: The fear that coffee and the caffeine it contains can cause heart disease, osteoporosis, infertility, or birth defects seems to be something designed to do little more than keep you awake at night worrying. But don't go chugging a carafe of coffee all by yourself. Common sense and moderation do have a place here. A coupla cups a day is AOK with us. Even three is not pushing the envelope—if it's filtered coffee. But if you're an espresso or French press aficionado, you should know that these unfiltered coffees do contain harmful compounds called terpenes, which may be the buggers that have been found to raise bad cholesterol levels in some coffee drinkers and increase the risk of a heart attack. Most of those tacky terpenes are filtered out from drip coffee.

Calling All Caffeine

Coffee may be one of the most concentrated sources of caffeine, but it's certainly not your only source. If caffeine puts you on edge (some of us get hyper, some of us don't), you should keep it to a bare minimum in your diet. Check out our caffeine chart to see where it might be lurking in your diet. Knowing just how much caffeine is there makes it easier to answer the question, "Coffee, tea, or me?"

What's New, What's True

Coffee may be the bearer of some good news for a change. Drinking coffee (and other caffeine-containing drinks) may work to boost your mood. Two big studies—the Nurses' Health Study and one done by a hospital group in California—showed that suicide rates were 50 percent lower in coffee drinkers. Whoa! Coffee as an anti-depressant? Researchers say that, as a matter of fact, the caffeine in coffee may act like a mild antidepressant. Nothing like a jolt of good news!

Source	Caffeine (milligrams)
Coffee, drip, 8 ounces	135
Coffee ice cream or frozen yogurt, 1 cup	30–85
Coffee, instant, 6 ounces with 1 teaspoon granules	57
Tea, leaf or bag, 8 ounces	50
Coffee yogurt, 8 ounces	45
Diet Coke, 12 ounces	45
Espresso, 1 ounce	40
Pepsi-Cola, 12 ounces	38
Coca-Cola Classic, 12 ounces	34
Vanilla Coke, 12 ounces	34
Snapple Peach Tea, 12 ounces	32
Chocolate bar, dark chocolate, 1.5-ounce bar	31
Tea, green, 8 ounces	30
Root beer, 12 ounces	22
Tea, instant, 8 ounces	15
Chocolate bar, milk chocolate, 1.5-ounce bar	10
Hot cocoa, 8 ounces	5

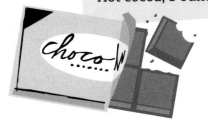

✳ Funky, Fabulous Food Facts

A cup of coffee can contain up to four times as much antioxidant activity as a cup of green tea! We kid you not. But it really shouldn't come as such a surprise. Coffee beans come from plants, and all plants produce phytonutrients.

Not Your Ordinary Joe

Looking for a healthy coffee alternative that still tastes and smells like the real thing? Have we got a coffee (sort of) for you! It's called Rocamojo and it's not coffee at all, but a roasted soy coffee alternative. Not only is it caffeine-free, it's certified organic and provides 6 grams of fiber, as well as B vitamins, iron, and a dash of calcium. And it actually tastes good. The only downside—it's not cheap and it's not calorie-free. A cup of Rocamojo provides about sixty calories, compared to a cup of black coffee, which is essentially calorie-free. If you don't want to totally let go of that real coffee taste, they also offer a fifty-fifty coffee/soy blend. No surprise then, that it contains caffeine and has half the calories, half the fiber, and half the nutrients of the 100 percent roasted soy drink. You can check out their website at *www.rocamojo.com.*

Tea

. . . .

Ancient Asian cultures must have instinctively known something about this brew that we only recently have learned: It's good for you. After all, they've been putting on the tea kettle for almost five thousand years! Okay. Fast forward to the present. While tea may be the second most popular beverage in the world, after water, most of it is enjoyed outside U.S. borders. We're slow to catch on, it seems, to the potential health benefits of drinking tea. Count 'em—less heart disease, less cancer, fewer cavities, stronger bones and last, but not least, possibly fewer pounds. And the latest news? Tea may help banish bad breath (halitosis for all you technical types). It seems that the natural phytonutrients in tea that provide all those other swell benefits also beat down the bacteria in your mouth that can make your breath stink. (Real attractive, eh?) Of course, this latest research was only in the lab, not in people's mouths, but as long as you're drinking tea for all its other health benefits, you might as well be aware of the latest possible plus about tea. However, bear in mind that even tea has a downside. Drink too much and you can stain your teeth. Teeth bleaching, anyone?

The Green Light for Weight Loss?

The burning tea question for all us weight-watching women, of course, is whether drinking green tea will help burn calories and knock off pounds. There are a gaggle of weight-loss supplements containing tea extracts that insist it's so. But when clearer heads prevail, the answer is, well, about as clear as mud. You've got your rat studies with those little rodents lapping up tea-laced water or getting injections of tea extract every day and you've got your human studies with volunteers dutifully taking daily supplements of tea extract. The bottom line? The studies seem to suggest that if you drink enough of the green stuff, you might be able to trigger a small increase (about 3 to 4 percent) in the number of calories you burn each day. And it may increase your body's ability to burn fat. Still, you can't brush aside the fact that the studies used tea extract supplements, not tea, and they studied only men and rodents (not that we're putting them in the same category). So is green tea worth a try? If you're willing to drink several cups of sugarless green tea a day,

* Funky, Fabulous Food Facts

Waiter, There's Green Tea in My Soup!

If you're on the prowl for another way to tuck some green tea into your diet, try this on for size. Next time you're in the mood for Japanese food, order ochazuke (oh-cha-zoo-KEH). It's basically rice topped with maybe salmon, vegetables, or seaweed (it's sort of the Japanese version of potluck—a great use of leftovers). The rice may be cooked and sitting in a soup of green tea or you may be called on to assemble some of the ingredients yourself at the table as part of the fun, and pour steaming hot green tea over the dish yourself. Teaism, a Japanese tea house and restaurant in Washington, D.C., actually gives diners written assembly instructions.

then we say, hey, why not? We're less enthusiastic about recommending supplements of tea extract. While there's no reason to believe they're bad for you, they're expensive and there's stronger proof that drinking the real thing is a healthy food choice.

The Other Tea

There's a new wrinkle in the tea tale. And it's a wrinkle you should welcome. It's white tea. No, it's not tea with milk. It's a relatively rare and pricey tea, whose fuzzy white buds are plucked from the same group of bushes as the tea leaves used to make green, black, and oolong teas. But *vive la différence*! It's clear to a light golden color and tastes clean and pure, yet still very tea-like. And no perfumey flavors, like some teas have. The real health kick is that, because it is minimally processed, it packs the same phytonutrient whollop as green tea, without the "green" taste, and it provides the same low level of caffeine.

✳ **Carolyn Says:** The first time I tasted or even heard of white tea was at The Dining Room of the Ritz-Carlton, Buckhead, in Atlanta. Chef Bruno Menard, who is dedicated to delighting his food savvy guests with new taste experiences, designed an après dinner tableside tea service. I could have chosen to mix in a little lavender honey, but the white tea has a natural sweetness and I was impressed with the subtle, yet complex flavors of the see-through brews. Then Bruno sent out a selection of teeny-tiny petit fours and the tea party continued!

Ice, Ice Baby!

Carolyn Says: There's nothing like a perfectly brewed iced tea poured into a tall glass. In fact, one of my tests of great restaurant service is how they brew and serve their iced tea. One of the most memorable iced tea moments happened during a lunch at Le Bec Fin, a very upscale restaurant in Philadelphia. I knew that the owner, Chef George Perrier, was infamous for demanding perfection, so I ordered iced tea with my lunch to see what would happen. It was an amazing peach-scented tea, not too perfumey, and brewed just right—not too weak, not too strong. The tall glass came with the proper long-handled iced tea spoon and I felt just as pampered as the folks at the next table who were being presented flutes of Champagne.

Milk

At 300 milligrams of calcium per eight-ounce glass, milk and calcium are like love and marriage, like a horse and carriage, like soup and sandwich—you get where we're going here. But milk has lost some of its respect as "nature's most perfect food" in the wake of controversies over drugs fed to dairy cows and the growing realization that a lot of people suffer from lactose intolerance (see our take on it on page 216). But don't toss the baby out with the bath water. Though the controversies over the effects of giving all those lactating cows hormones and antibiotics to keep them pumping out the white stuff is

Funky, Fabulous Food Facts

Raw milk sounds so earthy and real. Yeah, it's real all right. It can make you *real* sick. We've got a news flash for you: The reason Monsieur Louis Pasteur invented pasteurization way back in the 1860s was to make raw milk safe to drink. Straight from the cow, your chances are pretty darn high that milk contains disease-producing bacteria. No health boon there. In fact, drinking raw milk is such a health risk that several states have banned its sale. If you find it, skip it.

far from settled, you don't have to wait for final judgment. You can opt for organic dairy products now. The law requires that organic milk comes from cows that have not been given any drugs to boost their milk production or fed anything that was treated with pesticides. And if milk gives you gas, try one of the lactose-reduced or lactose-free products. Not only is milk one of the best calcium sources around, it's also an excellent source of vitamin D—one of those hard-to-come-by nutrients that will keep your bones hanging tough for years to come. (See chapter 3, The Dish on Superfoods, for the story on the added health benefits of fermented dairy products such as yogurt with live and active cultures.)

Milk Matters

Reduced-fat milk—contains 2 percent fat by weight; that comes out to about 42 calories from fat in an eight-ounce glass.

Low-fat milk—contains 1 percent fat by weight; that shakes out to about 21 calories from fat in an eight-ounce glass.

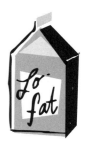

Skim milk—contains no fat.

Ultra What?

If you'd like to switch to skim, but just can't deal with the pale, bluish, watery-like appearance, you might want to give ultrapasteurized (UHT) milk a go. Because of the way it's processed, UHT skim milk has a creamier texture than regular skim, making it easier to sneak fat-free dairy in your diet. What about nutrition? The nutrient content is the same, with ultrapasteurized milk providing the same amount of calcium, potassium, and vitamins A, C, and D (which is added) as regular pasteurized milk.

Are You Really Allergic to Milk?

How often have you heard someone say, "I'm allergic to milk," but then you witness them eating a dish that contains milk without so much as a hiccup? They may not be able to drink a glass of milk without rumbling down below, but they are most certainly not allergic to milk. A true milk allergy is like an allergy to peanuts. It can be a life or death situation if you take in even a tiny amount. If drinking milk merely makes your stomach talk back or gives you sometimes painful cramps, then what you most likely have been saddled with is lactose-intolerance—which is a whole different can of worms. If you're allergic to milk, you're reacting to milk proteins and even a tiny amount can put the immune system on high alert and land you in the hospital. Lactose-intolerance, on the other hand, is your body's lack of ability to break down lactose, the natural sugar found in milk. A small amount of milk in a recipe probably won't bother you at all; even milk in your coffee and possibly a small amount of milk on your cereal will go unnoticed. But try downing an eight-ounce glass of milk and your bowels will let you know about it. Here's some dish on dairy if you have lactose-intolerance: Yogurt is low in lactose and the good bacteria it contains actually digest some of the lactose for you. Bottom line: Yogurt may be your best dairy decision. What are your odds of having either condition? About one out of every four people has lactose-intolerance; only about forty in ten thousand might have a milk allergy.

Got Soy Milk?

If soy milk is your "dairy" beverage of choice, there are a few soy stats you need to know:

* Some soy milks contain sugar, especially chocolate-flavored varieties.

* Unlike cow's milk, soy milk isn't a natural source of calcium. Look for a soy milk that's calcium- and vitamin D–fortified (boosts calcium absorption).

* Natural compounds in soy interfere with calcium. You'll need about 25 percent more calcium from soy milk than you would from cow's milk, to get the same benefit.

* Not all soy milks are organic. Read the label to be sure.

* Regular soy milk has about the same number of calories as regular cow's milk. Choose a lighter version to cut calories.

Sports Drinks

The dish on sports drinks is a one-liner: Unless you're a real athlete— marathoner, competitive tennis player, long-distance bicyclist, or perhaps you've got your sights set on the Women's Iron Man Triathalon in Hawaii next year—you probably don't need 'em. For all the rest of us weekend warriors or even five-times-a-week-to-the-gym crowd, water will most likely do you just fine. Even followers of Bikram yoga—that's the one where you subject yourself to saunalike conditions and sweat profusely while assuming yoga positions (don't ask)—should be able to get along with water alone—as long as you get some sodium from another source— maybe a snack with your water bottle. If, however, you fall into the ultrafit category or exercise intensely for more than an hour and a half at a stretch, then you'll need the extra boost of sodium, potassium, and calories that most sports drinks provide. On the other hand, nutritionists who do research for sports drink companies say sports drinks are for anyone who

✳ Party Hearty Last Night? Try a Sports Drink!

Carolyn Says: Rehydrating isn't just for sports fans anymore. If you had a bit too much to drink out on the town, pour yourself a sports drink before going to bed or first thing in the morning to aid in hangover recovery. Alcohol causes dehydration, which can bring on headaches and a foggy mind in the morning. So, forget the old maxim to reach for a bit of "hair of the dog" to cure what ails ya; the electrolytes and fluids in sports drinks will help get you back to feeling like your peppy self again.

exercises. Studies show that flavored sport drinks go down easier, so you're more likely to drink enough to rehydrate (replenish lost fluids) and replace electrolytes (sodium and potassium), plus they're more quickly absorbed and take care of your thirst in short order. And another recent study found that sports drinks don't make you go over your calorie quota for the day. You simply cut back later. Well, maybe, maybe not. Our guess is whether or not sports drinks become just another source for extra calories, rather than taking the place of calories you already get, is very much an individual thing.

Sports Drinks	Calories (per 8 ounces)
Ultima	16
Gatorade	50
AllSport	70
PowerAde	70
Met-RX	75
CytoMax	80
Accelerade	93
Endurox R4	187

✳ The Sports Drink Taste Challenge

Densie Says: I chatted with a good friend of mine, Kristine Clark, Ph.D., R.D., the director of Sports Nutrition at Penn State University, who also happens to be the nutritionist for the U.S. Women's Soccer Team (yeah, that women's soccer team) and an avid exerciser herself, about sports drinks. Though, with no irony in her voice whatsoever, she refers to herself as a "casual marathoner," I consider her one fit chick, who knows what she's talking about. At Penn State, she teaches sports nutrition, and every year does a nonscientific taste test with her students on which sports drink tastes the best. "Every year, hands down, it's the same. AllSport by Monarch Beverage Company comes out on top," she says. PowerAde and Gatorade are two more she recommends for taste and for energy. All three provide sodium and potassium and are within the range of carbs she recommends for refueling.

Send In the (Fruit) Smoothies

Don't ya just love the name? Smoothies. It sounds so soothing and good for you. So, how can something that sounds so light and healthy carry such a heavy calorie load? What started out as a great light idea—fresh fruit whipped into a froth and sucked through a straw—has gone the way of souped-up coffee drinks. (In fact, some of them *are* coffee drinks!) Heavy on the calories, and sometimes light on the fruit. A quick scan of smoothie selections uncovers calorie counts that range from about sixty-five to more than six hundred per serving. Every added ingredient, especially fat-happy ingredients like ice cream and whole milk, pushes the calorie count upward. Real fruit smoothies—read whipped fruit—are a great way to get several servings of fruit in one shot. But those add-ons (unless it's skim milk) do little more than add extra fat and calories. The best way to have your smoothie and eat it too? Get the smallest serving they have; most serve up about sixteen to twenty-two ounces a cup. If that's the smallest serving they offer, see if you can't persuade the kid behind the counter to give you a half serving. Eliminate half the temptation and you've already won half the battle. Or you could make smoothies at home. There are lots of smoothie recipes to be found on the Internet that are mouthwatering good (yes, Virginia, there is a *www.smoothie-central.com*), as well as some cookbooks devoted to nothing but smoothie recipes.

Potent Potables— How 'bout a drink?

Whether you're in the mood for a cold beer, a tall vodka and tonic, or a goblet of wine, all alcoholic beverages have one thing in common— they contain alcohol—but in widely varying amounts. So, even if you're choosing a light beer instead of hard liquor, it's important to know some basic alcohol equivalents. The USDA defines a "drink of alcohol" as twelve ounces of beer (regular or light) = 1½ ounces of 80-proof spirits = 5 ounces of wine. So, no matter what you're drinking, keep track based on what's called a "drink," not on how big the serving is or how tipsy you feel.

> Tell everyone to have a wonderful time and not to mix their drinks too much.
> —Julia Child

12 oz. = 1½ oz. = 5 oz.

Wine Appreciation 101

Of all the drinks, perhaps more has been written about wine—the culinary joys of drinking the fruit of the vine, and more recently the health properties it bestows—than any other beverage. Wine countries of the world, from France to Italy to Spain to Northern California and all the way down under to Western Australia, are among the most beautiful places on Earth, and the lifestyle of the people who live in wine-producing regions is to be envied. This is where, as friend and cookbook author Barbara Albright observes, "Winemakers are farmers working the land, but *these* are farmers with really good taste!" Roses tumble at the end of each row of grapevines, houses are filled with art and music, and blue jeans are worn with fine linen shirts. Parties are casual affairs with long tables of seasonally fresh foods surrounded by family and friends who come together to celebrate the bounty of life. Wine is enjoyed with meals and with respect. Wine is treated as a food matched with the menu. Wine is a state of mind and it's part of a lifestyle that embodies our motto to be healthy and fabulous! Don't be afraid of looking like a bumpkin if you don't know the best wine selection, the best way to hold your glass, or the best food to pair it with. Just taste and enjoy.

The Height of Food and Wine

One of the greatest ways to jump in and learn the secrets of the vine is to go to a wine festival. The Food & Wine Magazine Classic, held each year in Aspen, Colorado, is considered the ultimate setting to sample a world of wine, with tasting classes taught by big-name experts and the winemakers themselves. Each year in June an enthusiastic crowd of about five thousand fills the fashionable Rocky Mountain town to mingle with top chefs, take cooking classes, relax at multi-course dinners, and sip wines from all over the globe. Hang at The Little Nell Hotel or Hotel Jerome on this weekend, and chances are you'll be wining and dining right next to celebrity chefs ready to talk food trends and recipes! Isn't that Thomas Keller of Napa Valley's French Laundry sharing an al fresco lunch with Chef Mario Batali of New York? One word to the wise, though. When drinking alcohol at high altitudes, remember that one drink counts as three! Caroline Says: The thin air of Aspen is where I discovered the importance of drinking plenty of water during the day and mixing in many nonalcoholic "mocktails" at night. (Something to keep in mind for après ski imbibing too!) For more information on the Food & Wine Magazine Classic at Aspen visit *www.foodandwine.com*.

✳ Funky, Fabulous Food Facts

While the taste differences between a $20 bottle of vino and a $120 bottle from a four-star restaurant may be worlds apart, the calorie counts are remarkably similar. Check out the calorie counts for libations on page 230. The numbers hold for both low-brow and high-brow vintages.

A Few Words About Wine

Carolyn Says: The first time I heard, "This wine has a good finish," I thought, "Yes, in fact, I'm finished and would like another glass, please." It was my first introduction to the unique language of wine. Wine writers, winemakers, wine sellers, wine lovers all talk wine-speak—a lexicon just about everyone has heard but perhaps hasn't understood, such as "It's a dry wine," "It was a good year," or "It's got a lot of oak." I say, all you really need to know is, do you like the wine? The rest is an evolution of knowledge that should be fun to pick up over time. Let's face it. When you first heard the word "Prada," you didn't know why Prada shoes were so sought after; now you do—it's the quality and finesse in the making. Same goes for wine. To learn more about wine, go to wine tastings, sample wines by the glass at restaurants, and talk to friends about which wines they give the thumbs-up. And just because you didn't like one winery's Merlot, doesn't mean you won't like another label. You wouldn't expect all brands of salsa to taste the same, why would you expect wines from different wineries to be identical?

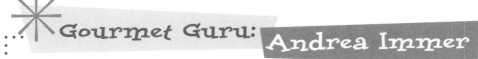

Gourmet Guru: Andrea Immer

Taste the Difference

Andrea Immer, master sommelier and author of *Great Wine Made Simple* (Broadway Books, 2000), suggests you get to know "The Big Six"—the six grapes that dominate wine-making—Riesling, Sauvignon Blanc, Chardonnay, Pinot Noir, Merlot, and Cabernet Sauvignon. Making it a group project is the best way to tackle a wine tasting. So, invite at least six friends over for the taste experiment and have some fun learning about wines. Andrea, who presents tastings to thousands of people each year, from beginners to experienced tasters, says, "When they taste these wines side by side at the same time, the reaction is always the same: Now I get it. Tasting these wines all together gives you the big picture—the whole spectrum of light, medium, and full body." Then, you can start getting into which wineries you like the most. You are on your way to becoming a wine expert too!

Champagne Wishes

How about a taste of the bubbly? If you say, "Fill my flute!" then you might be interested to know that champagne is actually one of the least caloric wine choices you can drink (80 to 90 calories per 4-ounce flute). But if you scream *no!* then maybe you've just had a bad experience with a lousy imitation. You know how bad you felt when you drank what you thought was champagne at your cousin's wedding? It was probably a cheap sparkling wine that was so sweet it went down fast, straight to your head, and left you with a sledgehammer pounding in your temples the next day. Waking up and realizing you really *did* wear that Scarlett O'Hara–style off-the-shoulder green taffeta bridesmaid dress, only made the hangover worse. Did you really carry that parasol? Oy *vey!* Next time, go for the good stuff.

> There comes a time in every woman's life when the only thing that helps is a glass of champagne.
>
> —Bette Davis in *Old Acquaintance* (1943). Amen!

Bubbly Basics: Recognizing the Real Thing

Sparkling wines, created from a blend of Chardonnay and Pinot Noir grapes, are made in most wine regions of the world from France to Spain to Australia and of course, Northern California's Napa Valley and Sonoma County. But only sparkling wines made in Champagne, a wine region of France, may be called "champagne." Other sparkling wines may be made the same way, called Methode Champenoise, but they may not use the champagne name on their labels.

Hip & Healthy Heroine: Mireille Guiliano

A Bubbly Lifestyle

The yellow label of Champagne Veuve Clicquot, made in the city of Reims in Champagne, is perhaps one of the most popular and sought-after sparkling wines today, because it's an icon of quality and style. Crisp, slightly spicy, perfect as an aperitif or with a meal, it's the "Armani of champagne." Mireille, who is President and CEO of Clicquot, Inc., lives in New York and travels back and forth to France just about every five weeks. She is one of our Hip & Healthy Heroines because she knows how to live with great energy and terrific style. Petite and full of life, she says, "I have never been on a diet!" Instead, she prefers to eat a light breakfast, such as yogurt, and enjoy small portions of delicious foods for lunch and dinner. Champagne is, of course, part of her healthy life too. She says, "Perhaps the best clue to unlocking the secrets of the health benefits of champagne are some real life examples. Madame Clicquot, who founded the company, lived to the elegant age of eighty-nine years (1777–1866). Currently we have four generations of Chefs de Caves or cellar masters from Champagne Veuve Clicquot still living. The oldest, M. Zeche, will turn one hundred next year and still swims almost every single day!" So, perhaps when Ponce de Leon was looking for the Fountain of Youth, he should have set his sights on Champagne!

The Dish Divas' Wine Rack

Great Whites

There's more to white wine than Chardonnay, although it is one of the most popular grapes for making wine, known for its big, buttery, lush, and full-bodied flavors. Other white grape varietals you should get to know include Chenin Blanc, Riesling, Sauvignon Blanc, Semillon, Pinot Blanc, Pinot Grigio and Viognier. Each of these wines has it own personality. Some are lighter, some are fruitier, some are more acidic;

sampling is the only way to tell which ones suit you. And it depends on what you're eating or where you are. For example, while dining al fresco on a hot summer day, a cool crisp glass of Sauvignon Blanc may be just the ticket. A roaring fire and roasted herb–stuffed chicken may be best matched with a creamy Chardonnay.

Karen MacNeil, author of *The Wine Bible* (Workman, 2001), says, "If Chardonnay can be compared to the sexy roundness of Marilyn Monroe, then Sauvignon Blanc is the polar opposite. More like Jamie Lee Curtis."

> *Wine is sure proof that God loves us and wants us to be happy.*
> —Benjamin Franklin

Meanwhile, there are wines with multiple personalities; some white and red wines will be elegant blends of two or even three different grapes. The blend will be indicated on the label.

Raise a Glass of Riesling

Riesling isn't the sweetie it used to be. In fact, dry Rieslings, with delicate refreshing flavors and less sweetness, are more popular today. (The term "dry" tips you off that a wine is less sweet.) Also worth noting, this wine is often low in alcohol and therefore lower in calories. Riesling can contain as little as 8 percent alcohol, while Chardonnays can be 13 percent or higher.

A Touch of Pink

From bright petunia pink to subtle shades of salmon, rosé wines are pretty in pink. And rosé wines are all the rage again, with many skilled winemakers creating their vineyard's version. Light and bright, they are wonderful paired with summer salads and pork tenderloin.

There are delicate and sought-after rosé sparkling wines too, but today's "pink champagne" is not as sweet as it used to be. And how cool can you be, *dahling*, standing at the bar, with a long flute full of pink sparkling in your hand, as you relax before your friends arrive.

But perhaps the most popular drink in pink is "white Zinfandel," made from red Zinfandel grapes with the skins removed. This wine is often mass-produced and is sugary, therefore a bit higher in calories.

Seeing Red

Red wines have gotten a lot of attention for being heart-healthy, and it's often a glass of red wine that's used to symbolize the connection between wine and health. All alcohol in moderation can boost heart health, see page TK, but the deep color of red wine is an indicator that this liquid is rich in phenols and other natural plant compounds that might pack an extra punch in disease prevention. So, let's learn our reds, shall we?

The biggest name in red wine and the heavy when it comes to dark colors and intense, full flavor, is Cabernet Sauvignon, which can range from bold and brash when young, to rich and satiny as it ages. The old term that "things mellow with age" certainly applies to red wines. Other reds to relish include Merlot, Syrah, Sangiovese, red Zinfandel, and Pinot Noir.

Pinot Envy

Of all the reds, Pinot Noir is the lightest—lightest in color and lightest in body. Wine expert Andrea Immer says it's her favorite red grape and describes it this way, "It's kind of like a red wine with a white wine texture. It's soft and feels like silk in your mouth." How's that for minimizing the intimidation factor with wine?!

Dessert Wines

How sweet it is! These are the real sugar daddies of the wine world. Clocking in at 18 percent alcohol (15.3 grams of alcohol in three ounces) and 128 to 138 calories per glass, dessert wines like port, sherry, or sauternes were made for sipping. That's why they are often served as a two- or three-ounce pour.

Here's to Your Health!

In a move that's sure to please wine lovers everywhere, the feds recently decided that winemakers could put information on labels suggesting there are health benefits to drinking wine. But they didn't take out all the stops. The labels aren't allowed to be so bold as to say "Wine is good for you," but they can direct wine drinkers to the government's Dietary Guidelines for Americans, which points out that wine and other alcoholic drinks can benefit your health, but that they can also carry health risks. So, there you have it; wine can be a mixed health blessing. It's not the carte blanche prescription for the fruit of the vine you were hoping for, perhaps. But read on.

Here's the dish: There's tons of research looking at the health effects of drinking not only wine, but beer and liquor as well. After debating the research for decades, most researchers have finally come around to admitting that yes, light to moderate drinkers (one to two drinks a day) have less risk of heart disease, the most common type of stroke, and are less likely to RIP at an early age than nondrinkers. It's even been called "the single best nonprescription way to prevent heart attacks." But—and here's the kick in the pants for us women—drinking appears to slightly increase the risk for breast cancer in younger women. It seems that drinking is most likely to provide health benefits to women over age fifty-five. So do you have to wait that long to enjoy a glass or two of your favorite vintage? That depends. If breast cancer runs in your family, then you may be doing more harm than good if you drink. But a glass of good wine, a gin and tonic with a twist, or a brewsky every now and again is one of life's little pleasures. Who are we to deny you that? Just be aware of the unanswered health questions surrounding younger women and alcohol, the next time you raise a toast to your health.

Beer

. . . .

If you listened to the hype, you'd think low-carb beer was the greatest dietary invention since, well, excuse the analogy, sliced bread. True, beer is brewed from hops, which is a grain, ergo beer is a source of carbohydrate calories. But even regular beer is not as loaded with carbs as you might think. A twelve-ounce regular beer provides somewhere in the neighborhood of 10 to 14 grams of carbs. Think that's a lot? Compare that to a single slice of whole-wheat bread, which provides about 18 grams of carbs. We have another little surprise for ya; so-called *"light" beers* are not that much lighter in carbs than *regular beers*—about 5 to 7 grams less. So there's really very little carb cutting, whether you're going from regular to *low-carb* or regular to "light" beers. If carbs are what you're trying to cut, you'd do just as well by cutting out a half slice of bread. Michelob Ultra, according to Anheuser-Busch, has the lowest carb count of any light beer with 2.6 grams per twelve-ounce serving. If you're a beer-drinking, low-carb gal, then your prayers have been answered. Miller Lite comes in a close second with 3.2 grams of carbohydrate. By the way, the level of alcohol is similar in regular, light, and low-carb beers, ranging from 4 to 5 percent. So, if you're counting carbs, go for the close up and make sure to read the beer bottle's label.

What about *nonalcoholic* beers? They have less than half a percent of alcohol and are designed for folks who want to drink with impunity. Ironically, they are even higher in carbs than regular beer, though the lack of alcohol still translates to fewer calories per bottle. That makes them a great "mocktail" choice at a cookout or a ballgame, if you are trying to cut calories and still want the taste of beer to wash down barbecue or that seventh-inning-stretch hot dog.

Beer Nutrition News

Okay, so here's the dish on beer, it might actually be good for you, with its folic acid and alcohol content and all. But another little known nutrition fact about beer is that it's a more-than-decent source of the mineral chromium (as much as 100 micrograms per 12 ounces). Why is that good news? Research shows that chromium can do amazing things when it comes to controlling your blood sugar. Lots of other foods contain small amounts of chromium, but nowhere near as much as some beers.

What's New, What's True?

Good nutrition makes a difference again! Folate, the B vitamin found in orange juice, leafy greens, and fortified breakfast cereals, may dampen alcohol's effect on breast cancer. A recent study done at the Harvard Medical School, published in the *Journal of the National Cancer Institute,* found that women who had at least one alcoholic drink a day were 89 percent less likely to develop breast cancer if they had high levels of folate in their blood, compared to those with the lowest blood levels. More good sources of folate: peas, beans, asparagus, cantaloupe, and papaya. How about a slice of cantaloupe with that cosmo?

Not All Calories Created Equal

Ever noticed that while you can down a few drinks and not notice a difference in your weight, the same number of calories in cheesecake, for example, can do a number on your waistline? It's not your imagination. It seems that your body isn't very fuel-efficient when it comes to the calories in wine, beer, and liquor. Translation: While alcohol provides 7 calories per gram, studies suggest that some of those calories are wasted before they can be stored as fat. The best news of all: Some studies have found that, in women, alcohol may actually be linked to weight loss. Now, before you embark on the "Wine Lover's

Diet," consider this: You're better off getting most of your calories from whole foods packed with vitamins, minerals, phytonutrients, and fiber, with the occasional libation as an added attraction.

But all this talk of wasting calories doesn't hold true for creamy concoctions like piña coladas and supersweet coffee and cream liqueurs. While the alcohol acts the same, the fat and sugar calories they contain count . . . big time. Check out the booze chart below to see how many calories you're getting altogether.

Alcohol by the Numbers

LIBATION	CALORIES
Piña colada (4½ ounces)	252
Crème de menthe (1½ ounces)	185
Screwdriver (7 ounces)	180
Coffee and crème liqueur (1½ ounce)	174
Margarita (5 ounces)	170
Beer (12 ounces)	150–198
Martini (2.5 ounce)	160
Rosé wine (5 ounces)	147
Dessert wine (3 ounces)	138
Port (3 ounces)	128
100-proof liquor (rum, gin, vodka, whiskey) (1½ ounces)	124
Bloody Mary (5 ounces)	118
Red wine (5 ounces)	106
White wine (5 ounces)	100
Light beer (12 ounces)	95–136
Champagne (4 ounces)	85

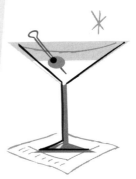

Cocktails

The glamour of cocktails is back in full swing at bars, restaurants, and chic parties. The martini glass is a sexy fashion accessory but, as the old saying goes, "One martini, two martini, three martini, floor!" Too much of a good thing is well, you know. And here's why—a 2½-ounce martini muscles into your system with 22 grams of alcohol, compared to 14 grams of alcohol in a 3½-ounce glass of Chardonnay. You can see why martinis can swiftly make you swoon.

✳ Funky, Fabulous Food Facts

Just in case you were wondering: A tablespoon of vanilla extract has as much alcohol as four ounces of beer.

✳ Cocktail Hour Calorie Saver

If you love rum and cola, vodka and tonic, or whiskey and ginger ale, you can save about 100 calories a drink if you choose a diet soft drink as your mixer. A rum and cola has 240 calories, while a rum and diet cola weighs in at 140 calories. So, if you like the flavor and you've decided you're okay with the artificial sweetener thing, then diet soft drinks can save you calories in your cocktails.

Cocktail Blues and Reds and Greens

All hail the creative cocktail concocter! With the competition fierce to impress customers who've "been there, drunk that," it's open season on daring drink designs. Whether you want vodka or gin, whiskey or rum, your drink can be any color of the rainbow or layers of colors with the addition of liqueurs and cordials.

Crème de menthe Midori turns it green, Grenadine red, Curaçao blue, Galliano yellow. And this stuff is powerful—most liqueurs and cordials are sixty to eighty proof. So, remember to count 150 to 190 calories for every sweet high-octane ounce and a half added to your cool cocktail.

At Blue Fin, the sleek eatery in New York's Times Square, they serve a blue martini aptly named the Blue Fin. For a color contrast and wild bit of whimsy, corporate beverage director Greg Harrington, of B. R. Guest restaurant group, tosses in an orange gummy fish. So your "what's-she-drinking?" cocktail ends up looking like a little aquarium in a martini glass. It'll make a real splash.

Blue Fin Cocktail

Greg Harrington, B. R. Guest Restaurants, New York

1 ounce Absolut Citron

2 ounces Hpnotiq Liqueur

½ ounce white cranberry juice

Red or orange gummy fish (optional)

1 Put the ingredients into a martini shaker.

2 Shake well and strain into a chilled martini glass. Add red or orange gummy fish.

Mocktails

Nonalcoholic drinks don't have to be party poopers. In fact, party hosts should plan on serving some just-as-festive mocktails for their guests who don't drink alcohol, who are the evening's designated drivers, and for smart partiers who know they'd better mix in a few hydrating beverages before calling it a night so they'll feel (and look!) better in the morning.

Sparkling bottled waters with a slice of lemon or lime are just the beginning. So, don't stop there. Whether you're out dancing the night away or dining al fresco with friends, the creative mocktail is our nonalcoholic drink of choice, because it's fun. No need to be a wallflower because the liquor's not flowing. Imagine you're at a bar with friends and everyone's having cosmos and margaritas or whatever and you tell the bartender, "I'll have a drink of water." Boring! Instead, look the bartender or waiter straight in the eye and smartly say, "I'll have a mocktail! Club soda, cranberry juice, with a twist of lime." It's sparkly

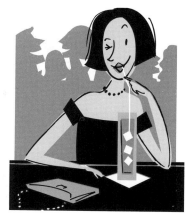

and rosy in a tall glass over ice and you still look like the life of the party. In fact, it will put more life into your party if you stay hydrated and limit your alcohol intake.

✳ Gourmet Guru: Dale DeGroff

Mastering the Mocktail

The cocktail king himself, Dale DeGroff, master mixologist and former head bartender at the legendary Rainbow Room, high atop Rockefeller Center in New York, has written a book, *The Craft of the Cocktail* (Clarkson Potter, 2002). **Carolyn Says:** I remember Dale preparing the perfect Manhattan for me once at the Rainbow Room bar when I was doing a CNN story on their sixtieth anniversary. The Rainbow Room has been serving glamour to guests since 1934. And as he poured the golden red liquid into the martini glass, the view from sixty-five stories up was a glorious sunset splashing that same amber color over the skyline of New York. Dale says, "Sadly, many bartenders don't want to encourage nonalcoholic drinks and will just offer juice or soda, but if you find a bartender who is passionate about his trade, he will embrace the challenge." A good way to proceed is to ask the bartender if he can concoct a fresh juice nonalcoholic cocktail for you. Let him experiment.

Here are two Marvelous Mocktail recipes from Dale. The orange and grapefruit juices add a healthy dose of good nutrition.

Grapefruit Julep

Dale DeGroff, aka King Cocktail, New York

The ingredients in this signature beverage combine to create a uniquely sweet burst of tropical fruit flavor.

2 mint sprigs

½ ounce lime juice

1 ounce honey syrup

5 ounces grapefruit juice

1 ounce pomegranate juice

1 Bruise one mint sprig in the bottom of a mixing glass with the lime and honey syrup.

2 Add the juices and shake. Strain over ice into a chilled rocks glass. Garnish with the remaining mint.

Sunshine Punch

Wedding showers, summer parties, and outdoor gatherings are the perfect occasions for this tropical, refreshing, fruity beverage. And if the taste of this cocktail isn't enough, the spiral lemon-rind garnish is sure to open your eyes.

2 ounces ruby red grapefruit juice

2 ounces orange juice

1 ounce pineapple juice

¼ ounce fresh lime juice

½ ounce simple syrup (equal parts honey and water)

½ ounce grenadine

Long lemon zest spiral

1 Cut a long spiral of lemon zest and prepare a tall glass with the lemon zest spiraling down to the bottom of the glass with ice holding it in place.

2 Shake all the ingredients well with ice and strain into the prepared glass.

✳ More Mocktails

Densie Says: Looking for more ideas for mocktails? How about a Funky Monkey or a Hot Fluffermutter? Intrigued yet? Check out *The Ultimate Liquor-Free Drink Guide*, by Sharon Tyler Herbst (Broadway Books, 2002).

✳ The Quaffer's Quiz

Susan Burke, registered dietitian extraordinaire and director of nutrition services for *www.eDiets.com*, helps visitors to this terrific online diet and nutrition website keep up-to-date and on-track in their quest to eat, drink, and be healthy. Put yourself to the test with her Quaffer's Quiz about alcohol and your health. And for more up-to-the-minute nutrition info and diet support, check out the website. Tell Susan the Dish Divas sent ya.

True or False

1 Alcohol is a stimulant.

2 If you eat before you drink, you won't get drunk.

3 Men and women handle alcohol the same.

4 White wine is a good choice if you want a drink with less alcohol.

5 Light beer has less of a kick than regular beer.

6 As long as you average a drink or two a day, it doesn't matter how much you drink on any given night on the town.

7 Red wine is the healthiest of all alcohol choices.

Look Out Below:

1 *False!* You may feel energized after that first drink, but the fact is, alcohol is a drug that acts as a depressant, like a tranquilizer or a sleeping pill, and it can lead to an unattractive lack of coordination and personality changes (and not usually for the better). Remember, alcohol in moderation is okay, but it's ultimately a gamble—the more you drink, the higher the health stakes.

2 *False!* Food doesn't prevent alcohol from being absorbed, but it does slow it down. The result: That drink "goes to your head" more slowly; the alcohol still gets there, just at a slower pace.

3 *False!* Alcohol has more of an effect on us women than men. Why? As women, we tend to be smaller and have less body water, so drink for drink, we tend to develop higher blood concentrations of alcohol and get tipsy quicker (and fail the breathalyzer test earlier in the evening) than a man who drinks the same amount.

4 *False!* A 5-ounce glass of wine has as much alcohol as a 1.5-ounce shot of eighty-proof spirits or one 12-ounce beer. So, a glass of wine, or a bottle of beer, for that matter, will have the same effect as a straight shot of scotch.

5 *False!* Light beers have slightly less alcohol and fewer calories. But while the calories may be one-third lower, there's actually little difference in alcohol content. What light beers dish up is a weak-flavored, lower-calorie beer with almost the same alcohol kick as regular beer.

6 *False!* The health benefits of alcohol are linked with one to two drinks a day. They can't be "saved up" over time and consumed in a one-day, party-hearty, let 'er rip binge. Some experts consider more than three drinks in one sitting to be binge drinking. And binges do more harm than good; they can cause your blood pressure to soar, not to mention unleash a deadly decline in your driving skills!

7 *False!* While it's true that substances in red wine, such as polyphenols and flavonoids that come from grape skins, are heart-healthy (polyphenols help promote healthy blood vessels and flavonoids are strong antioxidants, which protect our cells from damage), better health and longer life are linked with moderate consumption of *all* kinds of alcohol. Even beer contains B vitamins that may aid in prevention of heart disease.

How'd Ya Do?

1–2 You may not be maximizing the health benefits of alcohol and avoiding its pitfalls. Go back and sip on the info in the answers.

3–4 Review and impress your friends with your alcohol and health know-how.

5–7 Cheers! *Prost! Salud! À votre santé!* To your potent potable prowess!

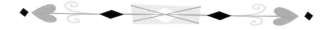

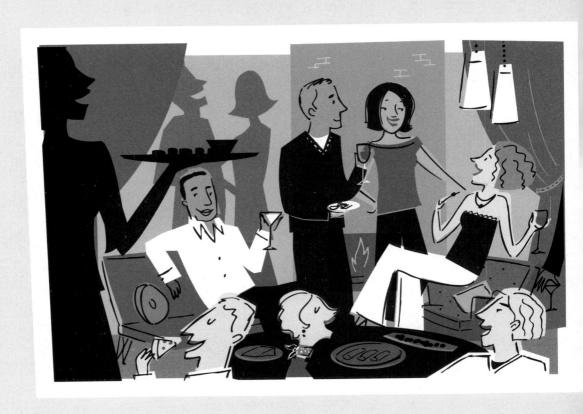

7 The Dish on Entertaining

Since the whole point of looking and feeling fabulous is to experience a little *joie de vivre*, let's throw a party! Entertaining at home—whether it's for cocktails, a cookout, or a buffet bash to watch a TV season finale—is a smashing way to demo your delicious newfound food philosophy. *The more you know, the more you can eat!* And now *you* know that eating healthy foods *does* mean saying yes to make-your-own-pizza parties or canapés with cocktails, as long as you offer the right ingredients. Plenty of veggies for the pizza, easy on the cheese. A nice assortment of party snacks from tasty bites of seared tuna, to baby carrots served with cucumber raita, a traditional Greek yogurt dip.

But just as you don't need to reveal the super-sale price on your new pleated mini, or just how often you get your highlights done, you don't have to announce your menu is "good-for-you." In fact, culinary icon and superexperienced party giver Julia Child recommends, "If you serve a health-conscious meal to guests, don't say so. Don't mention it

> My doctor told me to stop having intimate dinners for four, unless there are three other people.
> —Orson Welles

239

at all. You shouldn't let nutrition get in the way of planning a good meal. Think taste first!"

Absolutely! So, as the Dish Divas, in this chapter we'll show you how to lay out a delicious spread that doesn't lead to midriff spread, while maximizing the pleasures of the table for everyone invited. Here's to the healthy high life! You'll garner great reviews on your food and your form! And to help you keep your cool in the kitchen, we've got some party-planning tips from the shopping to the chopping. So, let's get the party started.

It's Your Party

Having fun with friends may be all about spontaneous good times, but when it comes to throwing a successful party, the experts say, "Plan, baby, plan!" Start with a theme—fancy or fancy-free? The number of guests—six friends for a brunch or sixty for a bash? And party pro Tony Conway, who owns Legendary Events catering company in Atlanta (and fifteen tuxedos), says, "I believe in invitations. It gives guests something to post and read and shows you didn't just throw it together." He assures us that there's no need to bust the budget on fancy printed invites. "The computer does it all today! Or send an e-vite. Make sure it shows the feel of the party so they know what to expect." Is it a clambake? Oh, I'm allergic to clams. What should I wear? Who wants to arrive at a seventies' party dressed for a Hawaiian luau? Actually that just might work!

Once you've got the wheels in motion, choose the menu. Tony says, "This will help you figure out when to shop, what to make ahead of time, what to buy already prepared, and what to do the day of the party. Need help? What are best friends for? Open one bottle of champagne early."

Party Talk with Tony

BTW—we asked and Tony did the math. In the past six years he's organized 2,400 parties. (He *must* be the go-to guy for hangover cures.) Tony is definitely a solid source of how to prevent festivity fiascos, so let's listen up. "Candles are lovely and my guests adore them. But be careful! Flowing jackets or dresses, scarves or sleeves can catch in the flames. Fill your fireplace with candles or put them anywhere out of traffic flow. I've had flowers in centerpieces catch on fire too. Flaming drinks are fun, not flaming dining room tables."

Another party pooper—running out of food! Tony says, "If you're setting up a buffet, it's best to have fewer items and plenty of backup, than ten different dishes and no refills. It's easier to manage too. And this may not be the fun part of partying, but you've got to plan for clearing. If everyone's in the kitchen, where are you going to put the dirty dishes?"

One solution—serve dessert in another room. If the chocolate truffles call, the crowd will follow and clear out of the kitchen to settle down in the den. But keep a few truffles stashed in the kitchen for those you-gotta-love-'em friends who like to lend a hand with the dishes. Be sure to mention that they're burning extra calories while they sample the sweets. Oh, you're such a genius!

Everybody's in the Kitchen

You don't need a big-bucks gourmet kitchen to entertain in style, but you do need to get things organized so you can cook for a crowd. Designing dream kitchens of all sizes (and for all budgets) makes Jan Walters happy. As the director of the Insperience Studio in Atlanta, she helps customers "test drive" KitchenAid and Whirlpool appliances in their showroom kitchens. Some are ultramodern, some have traditional charm, but all of the kitchens inspire you to get in there and cook! It's kind of like going to an auto dealer showroom and imagining yourself behind the wheel. "Try it, you'll like it" is apparently all the rage in the kitchen biz today. The Viking Range Corporation has eight Culinary Arts Centers nationwide; you can get to know their high-performance appliances by taking cooking classes with chefs and cookbook authors. Go to *www.vikingrange.com.*

And while working over a hot stove is still the best way to get a meal on the table, kitchens today are also "hot" in a fashion sense. (That classic KitchenAid stand mixer even comes in thirty-two pick-your-personality colors now, from tangerine to lavender.) Jan Walters says it's all about casual entertaining today. "The formal dining room is disappearing. Kitchens are designed to be open and be connected with living spaces. If everyone ends up in the kitchen you don't want it all boxed in. That makes clutter-control important, with plenty of easy-to-access storage." Guests should see you calmly cooking, not spilling salad dressing all over a month's worth of mail piled up on the counter.

But no matter how sleek and trendy kitchens become (we saw a double-sided KitchenAid refrigerator with mirrored door fronts—talk about a deterrent to raiding the fridge!), the basic laws of design don't change. If you're thinking of redesigning your personal cooking space, Jan reminds us of the rules. "No matter how big or small, an efficient kitchen respects the work triangle. That's the flow between the sink, the refrigerator, and the stove. If guests get in the way there, it can really slow things down." That's where the island or peninsula comes into play and no, we're not talking about going to the beach. These countertop options help define work areas. You stay on your side of the island and I'll stay on mine!

But Jan suggests, "For people who want their friends to pitch in, it's really helpful to have two prep areas with sinks." Hey, two sinks is the way to go when sharing a bathroom, isn't it? Check out *www.kitchenaid.com* to shop for more dream kitchen ideas.

Hip & Healthy Heroine: Barbara Fairchild

Less Is Always More

As the editor in chief of *Bon Appétit* magazine, Barbara Fairchild plans real-life parties, from patio dinners at her home in Los Angeles to events for hundreds in New York's hot hotels. Let's just say she knows how to coach you through the highpoints and hassles of hosting. Here are some of Barb's tips:

- ✳ Compose a menu of as many do-ahead dishes as possible, or do as many steps ahead of time as you can. Three courses are plenty: appetizer, main, dessert.

- ✳ Supplement with store-bought items; this is common practice today and there is so much excellent food out there now: great olives and roasted nuts for a simpler appetizer time, precut crudités with salsa, etc., fantastic breads to pass alongside the main course, those kinds of things.

- ✳ Look at your schedule objectively to assess what you can really get done and when.

- ✳ Set the table the night before, if necessary, adding the flower arrangement on the afternoon of the party.

- ✳ Set out serving plates and bowls ahead of time with Post-it notes of the designated dishes inside.

- ✳ Tape a copy of the menu to the refrigerator so that you can refer to it as you go along. Similarly, attach the recipe to the refrigerator as you are working on it. Then make a quick checklist of what needs to be finished right before guests arrive.

- ✳ Don't forget to put on your mascara!

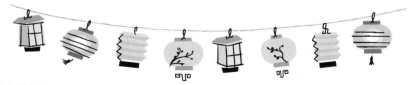

Hip & Healthy Heroine: Joy Sterling

A Movable Feast

Some of the best parties, planned by the most thoughtful hosts, keep the meal in motion. Why sit in one room, when you can start in the garden, move indoors, and end up in front of the fire? All that getting up and down and walking around is good for your digestion, too. Plan a walk before or after the meal around the block, down to the beach, or through the park, and you've got some low-impact, high-interest fitness to match your menu. One of the ultimate settings for this kind of entertaining is California's wine country. Joy Sterling, of Iron Horse Ranch and Vineyards, likes to entertain guests with a four-course "lunch and learn" at her family's Sonoma County winery. It starts with a flute of bubbly at the winery overlooking the vineyard's vista below, where fruit trees and poppies add even more natural decoration to the acres of Pinot Noir and Chardonnay grapes that go into the Iron Horse sparkling wines. "Our grapes are all hand-harvested. It's like a rosebush; some clusters mature while others are still buds. And there's no big assembly line here. Each bottle gets a personal touch." And that's what you see on your walk down the hill to the building where the bottles are kept and corked. Then it's on up the hill to a house built in 1876, where Joy's parents, Audrey and Barry, live and welcome their guests for their traditional harvest lunches.

Now it's through the house filled with art from world travels, past the dining room table festooned with a long line of crystal candlesticks, and into the back garden where more sparkling wine awaits. Chef Christopher Greenwald knows the Sterlings like big flavors but small courses of healthy fare. After fresh sardines served with yellow and red cherry tomatoes paired with Cuvee R (a blend of Sauvignon Blanc and Viognier), we taste fried green tomatoes with a peppery buttermilk sauce and then a main course of grilled squab jazzed up with a hot and sweet chile jam paired with Iron Horse Chardonnay. After just enough homemade ice cream with fruit, it's time to move again for tea in the garden. There's even a whimsical "flower bed"—a white wrought iron bed in the middle of the foliage—where Barry Sterling likes to take his afternoon naps. So great food, great wine, a mobile feast, and a nod toward the value of meditating in nature to melt away the stress of deciding when to pick the grapes!

Party Noshes

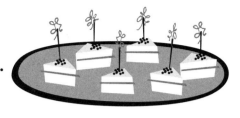

No matter what you plan to serve the gang, what's a get-together without a party snack spread? Just keep in mind how easy it can be to gobble down hundreds of calories before dinner even hits the plate. So, here are some ball-park figures for some common munchies.

The Cost in Calories

Baguette (2¼-inch slice)	75
Baked potato chips (1 ounce—11 chips)	120
Camembert (1 ounce)	90
Caviar (1 tablespoon)	40
Cheese crackers, bite-size (1 ounce)	150
Chex party mix (1 ounce)	130
Cream cheese (1 tablespoon)	50
Egg rolls, appetizer (1 roll)	40
Goat cheese (1 ounce)	70
Guacamole dip (1 tablespoon)	40
Herb garlic cheese spread (1 tablespoon)	35–70
Jarlsberg cheese (1 ounce)	100
Nuts (1 ounce)	160–200
Olives, all varieties (2)	10–40
Olive salad (⅓ cup)	40
Pâté de foie gras (1 tablespoon)	60
Potato chips (1 ounce—20 chips)	150
Pretzels (1 ounce)	110
Salsa (1 tablespoon)	5
Smoked salmon (1 ounce)	33
Sour cream dip (1 tablespoon)	25
Table water crackers (5 crackers)	70
Tortilla chips (1 ounce—17 chips)	110
Triscuit crackers (7 crackers)	120

✳ For an amazingly thorough source of nutrition info on cheeses, olives, spreads, and breads, check out *www.wegmans.com*.

Entertain More? That's a Laugh!

Before you break out the good china and clear that pile of bills off the dining room table, make sure you've got some funny friends on the guest list. Sharing a meal and a yuk or two has actually been proven to boost your health big time. So keep the jokes flowing with the festivities! Researchers in Japan found that laughing during a meal helped reduce postmeal blood sugar levels (which helps protect against diabetes and its complications, such as heart disease). They think it's because laughter increases energy consumption by working abdominal muscles and might affect the endocrine system, which controls blood sugar. Laughter is also linked to improved blood circulation and helps boost the immune system. Miss Manners always said don't discuss serious stuff like politics or religion over dinner. Keep it light and make entertaining a laughing matter! So, there were these two guys sitting at a bar . . .

What a Coincidence: Healthy Is "In"

Menus with a variety of tastes, textures, and colors are simply the best, no matter what your theme might be. And it turns out that's the perfect scenario for offering healthy foods. Bright notes of citrus in the salad, smooth soups of winter squash, and entrées happily surrounded by vibrant vegetables all look great, taste great, and happen to be great for you. Caterer Tony Conway says if guests have a delicious meal that doesn't weigh them down, they're happy to be there. "We do lots of fish. Whole roasted fish can be beautiful. I use a lot of peppers in dishes today. Bold flavors, but not too hot. Risottos with vegetables are popular. And stacked salads can be real show stoppers, stacking multicolored tomatoes or beets with mozzarella or goat's milk cheeses."

Gourmet Guru: Anne Quatrano

Annie's Awesome Arugula

Carolyn Says: Sometimes you taste a dish and know you will always remember the moment. These are the inspiring foods and flavors you want to try to collect and re-create at home. Here's one of those food memories for me. I was dining with some girlfriends at the very hip and *moderne* Floataway Café in Atlanta, owned by chefs Annie Quatrano and Clifford Harrison. Everyone ordered something different to taste test as much as possible from the wonderfully creative menu. Marinated Georgia coast shrimp with pickled red onions. Organic zucchini and crookneck squash drizzled with truffle oil on paper-thin and crusty pizzas. I ordered an arugula salad. When my dish came to the table I looked at it and was a bit disappointed—it was a pile of leaves. My friends offered, "Want to try ours?" I gave the salad a chance and woah! This was the best pile of leaves I had ever tasted. The arugula was peppery with a fresh crunch and the dressing was a brilliant yet simple mix of lemon, olive oil, sea salt, and black pepper.

This salad didn't need croutons, or Parmesan cheese curls, or tomatoes for color. The arugula spoke of the fresh green earth and the expert vinaigrette livened up its language. The secret's in the sauce, as they say.

Here's **Annie's Awesome Arugula** in her own words, "The salad is dressed with a squeeze of lemon, a fruity Tuscan extra-virgin olive oil, sea salt, and cracked black pepper. For one salad, about 3 ounces of arugula—of course, the arugula was fresh, local, and organic—1 half-lemon squeeze into a bowl, about 1 teaspoon of olive oil, and salt and pepper to taste." Toss and wow your guests.

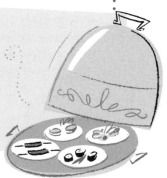

Party "'Round the World"

Barbara Fairchild of *Bon Appétit* magazine says American cooks are more adventurous in their tastes now, and she thinks that's just great. Party givers can really run with an international idea these days and not have to worry about whether a menu might be too foreign for guests. The more authentic the recipe, often the healthier the dish will be. Embrace true regional Italian and French cooking, authentic Mexican food, Moroccan spicing, and all sorts of Asian, from Thai to Vietnamese. And the best part? You don't have to shop till you drop to find the right ingredients. Supermarkets are advancing these culinary travels by offering a record number of fresh and packaged ethnic ingredients. It all adds up to a global revolution in home entertaining.

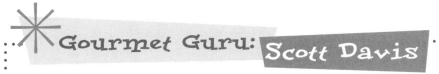

Gourmet Guru: Scott Davis

Money Can Buy You Loaves

No time to bake brioche before the brunch? Scratch the idea and leave it to a team of experts. Corner bakeries (family-owned or multiunit megastores) now dot the urban landscape. And even though millions of folks are on carb-control, there's never been a better time to buy excellent quality breads. Still, we thought it best to turn to an expert for advice. From three-cheese semolina to kalamata olives, master baker Scott Davis of Panera Bread, a Missouri-based company with more than 500 bakeries around the country, knows dough. "Look for handcrafted breads made by skilled bakers. Bread is a living organism and you bake it differently, depending on heat and humidity. Quality shows in the crust with nuances of aroma and texture."

He encourages everyone to buy bread whole, not sliced, so the crust keeps moisture in as a natural packaging. "Plastic wrap is a bad idea. It causes moisture to collect on the crust. Instead, just slice off what you need and set the loaf on its end." Use leftovers to make croutons or mix into salads. That's what the Italians do when making panzanella salad! Scott even encourages you to think of food and bread pairings, like you would with wine. That's the reason dark brown German ryes go so well with bratwurst and subtle yet crunchy French baguettes are happy with strong-flavored cheeses, such as Camembert or Brie. If you're cutting back on the amount of bread you eat, that's all the more reason to make sure you bring home the best.

It's a Breeze If You Braise

Cooking everything at the last minute often requires eight arms and sixteen sauté pans, so choosing a main course that's braised is often the smart way to go. From beef stews to coq au vin (chicken in red wine) and osso buco (veal shanks in white wine), braising means cooking in liquid for a long period of time. It's also a good choice for lean cuts of meat because the slow cooking tenderizes protein fibers by gently breaking them down. And because most of the work is done hours ahead of your dinner, braising helps prevent party host breakdown too. All you have to do is lift the lid and let the aromas waft toward the dining room. Gerry Klaskala, chef and owner of Aria Restaurant in Atlanta, loves the depth of flavors in slow-cooked dishes. Aria may be oh-so-modern as you enter through a curtain of stainless steel beads, but Gerry's recipe for braised lamb shanks is a timeless classic.

Sauvignon Blanc Braised Lamb Shanks

Gerry Klaskala, Executive Chef, Aria Restaurant, Atlanta

YIELD: *8 servings*

2 tablespoons olive oil

8 lamb shanks (bone in and fat trimmed)

Kosher salt

Ground black pepper

2 onions, peeled and cut into large dice

2 carrots, peeled and cut into large dice

2 celery stalks, cut into large dice

1 leek, white part, cut into large dice

4 fresh tomatoes, diced

12 garlic cloves

6 sprigs thyme

3 sprigs rosemary

2 cups Sauvignon Blanc or another crisp, acidic white wine

Chicken stock to cover shanks, about 2 quarts

For sauce:

1 tablespoon all-purpose flour

1 tablespoon milk

½ cup small diced carrots

½ cup small diced celery

2 tablespoons chopped parsley

1 Heat the olive oil in a large roasting pan with a lid.

2 Season the lamb shanks generously with salt and pepper.

3 Sear the lamb on all sides until lightly brown. Remove and set aside. Remove all but 1 tablespoon of the oil.

4 Add the vegetables, garlic, thyme, and rosemary. Cook until lightly browned.

5   Add the wine and reduce by half.

6   Add the lamb back to the pan and cover with the chicken stock. Bring to a simmer, cover, and cook in a preheated 350 degrees F oven for 2½ to 3 hours or until quite tender.

7   Remove all the fat from the top of the braising liquid. Set aside the lamb shanks and keep warm. Strain the liquid. Put the liquid back in pan over medium-high heat.

8   Mix together the flour and milk to form a slurry. Whisk the slurry into the liquid. Reduce the liquid to a sauce consistency.

9   Before serving, add ½ cup each diced carrot and diced celery and 2 tablespoons chopped parsley to the sauce, and heat until the vegetables soften, about 20 minutes.

10 Serve one lamb shank per person. Ladle the sauce over the lamb and serve with either polenta or couscous and blanched haricots verts. Garnish with fresh parsley.

Recipe note: Gerry suggests starting this recipe the day before or the morning of your party, so the braising liquid can be cooled and you can skim the excess fat from the top. It keeps the lamb shanks tender and juicy too. If making ahead, stop after step 6 above. Then before dinner start with step 7 and add the lamb shanks to the sauce to reheat while the vegetables are softening.

Wine note: Gerry suggests a lighter style red such as Sangiovese.

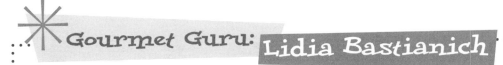

Gourmet Guru: Lidia Bastianich

Eat Your Vegetables Italian-Style

Are you getting bored with the same old steamed broccoli and boiled new potatoes? Then leave the country. A trip to Italy (or a great Italian restaurant at home) will awaken your taste buds with the lively flavors of the Mediterranean. Lidia Bastianich is the ultimate gourmet guide to Italian cooking as co-owner of three New York City restaurants—Felidia, Becco, and Esca, author of three cookbooks, host of two public television series, and at least once a year she leads culinary tours through Italy. Carolyn Says: When I joined Lidia in Tuscany, she had taken over the kitchen of a wonderful villa in the middle of a vineyard to teach an enthusiastic American bunch who signed up to experience Italy via a cooking school vacation. Classroom projects happily turned into lunch as we gathered on the terrace to discuss life, love, and the pursuit of fabulous food. On this day, Lidia included a lesson on cooking and eating artichokes. Her recipe for braising them takes artichokes to a new flavor level. You'll never cook them in plain water again!

Suggested reading: Lidia's Italian-American Kitchen (Knopf, 2003).

How to Eat an Artichoke

Artichoke eating is a ceremony of sorts, a step-by-step finger food that helps reinforce your newly discovered satisfaction of eating slowly. Tear off one leaf at a time. Pull the leaf through your teeth to scrape off the tender bits. Enjoy one after the other, dipping into the braising liquid. When you get to the meaty heart in the middle, remove the bristly stuff—so you don't choke on your 'choke—and savor the best part of all!

You'll-Think-You're-in-Tuscany Braised Artichokes

Lidia Bastianich, Restaurant Felidia, New York

YIELD: *4 servings*

Juice of 1 lemon

6 garlic cloves

4 large but tender artichokes with stems, one per person

2 tablespoons olive oil

2 tablespoons butter

2 tablespoons chopped parsley

1 tablespoon chopped mint

4 small whole dried peperoncino peppers or 1 teaspoon crushed

1 teaspoon salt

2 cups good vegetable or chicken stock

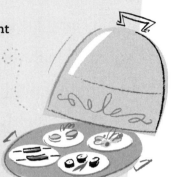

1   Cut the lemon and squeeze the lemon juice into 1 quart of water.

2   With a sharp paring knife, pull off the tough outside leaves of the artichokes, proceeding from the bottom to the top and cutting off the top third.

3   Peel the stem and place the artichoke in the lemon water. Keep in lemon water until you finish cleaning all the artichokes. Remove the artichokes from the water, drain them well, and pat them dry with a towel.

4   In a deep pan, where the artichokes fit snugly, set them with their stems up. Add all the remaining ingredients and bring to boil. Let them simmer for 30 minutes, covered, then serve in a soup plate with the juices from the pan.

Presentation Is Everything

Okay, so you're sold on serving smaller portions in a parade of tasty courses. But don't play it safe at the plate. Mix up the shape and size of your serving pieces. Pretty teacups are perfect for serving soups. Hollowed-out orange halves can display the citrus sorbet. Or use long-handled iced-tea spoons to present tiny bites of tuna arranged on a platter. (Just don't get too creative and start grabbing artsy platters off the walls. Dishes that say "for decoration only" on the back are not to be used for serving food because they can contain lead-based paints!)

Three-Martini Lunch

All this talk about multipurpose plating segues nicely to the always elegant martini glass. Gina Christman, publisher of *Atlanta Homes & Lifestyles* magazine, collects these long-stemmed beauties in all kinds of designs—from basic to bejeweled. At her casually glamorous gatherings, they're the perfect size to sport more than vodka and gin. How about these party players presented in a martini glass?

One martini: Cold soups to sip

Two martini: Shrimp as finger food

Three martini: Frozen dessert to delicately spoon

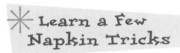

Learn a Few Napkin Tricks

Densie Says: One of the easiest ways to add a touch of class to your table is to have an elegantly folded napkin at each place setting. It's a guaranteed conversation piece and some of the basic napkin tricks are incredibly easy. You just need some good-quality, colorful napkins and a set of instructions. For starters, check out *www.freenapkinfolding.com.*

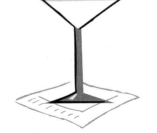

You're Going to Put That Eggplant Where?

Flowers can be expensive, so why not dip into the vegetable bin to come up with a creative centerpiece? Napa Valley winemaker and uber-entertainer Molly Chappellet champions this edible decorating idea in her book *A Vineyard Garden* (Viking Penguin, 1991), and we still love it! Everyone knows you can put a pumpkin on the table in October, but Molly goes way beyond that with broccoli forests and piles of golden peppers. She believes in elevating the beauty of fresh produce to art, and nothing goes to waste. "Tomorrow, you can dine on broccoli soufflé and golden pepper soup!"

Trade Ya!

Carolyn Says: Don't know where to find party recipes "sure to please"? Some of the best dishes I know are ones I've discovered through friends. You go to a party and say "Wow! This is really delicious. I'd love to have your recipe!" It's the ultimate cooking compliment. You've sampled it and you know it can't be that impossible to re-create—after all a friend made it, not a team of chefs. My friend and food writer Elizabeth McDonald brought this angel hair pasta dish to a potluck meeting of Les Dames d'Escoffier in Atlanta. (Les Dames is an international organization of women with professions in the food world.) Now, the recipe is from her husband Rob's Italian family, but she made it! I love the surprise of bright citrus notes with aromatic rosemary. The flavors are so forward that you're satisfied with pasta portion control! Your guests may ask for Rob's recipe too.

Rosemary Lemon-Lime Pasta

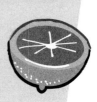

Rob McDonald, terrific cook and photographer, Atlanta

YIELD: *8 servings*

¾ cup extra-virgin olive oil

1 cup grated Parmesan cheese

¼ cup minced fresh rosemary

Juice of 2 lemons and 1 lime

Salt and freshly ground pepper to taste

1 pound dried pasta (I used angel hair. I bet some fresh pasta would also be fabulous!)

1 In a large bowl, combine olive oil, cheese, rosemary, lemon and lime juices. Add the salt and pepper and stir to blend.

2 Meanwhile, cook the pasta in a large pot of salted water until al dente. Drain well and add to the bowl of sauce, toss to coat, and serve at once.

Gourmet Guru: Chef Mario Batali

Party Pasta Tip

Ya can't miss him! Chef Mario Batali wears bright orange high-top sneakers and khaki shorts, even in the winter, so he always looks like he's having fun in the kitchen. And Mario wants you to have a great time cooking Italian food too. Owner of Babbo and several other Italian eateries on the "it" list in Manhattan, Mario shares his culinary soul through recipes in cookbooks, TV shows, and cooking classes. **Carolyn Says:** Pasta is a perennial party favorite and one of the simple, yet brilliant tips I learned from Mario comes into play after you've boiled your pasta. During a cooking class at the Food & Wine Magazine Classic in Aspen he announced to the eager crowd of sophisticated foodies, "Don't drain all of the water away! Pasta water is your friend. It adds flavor and a little bit of starch for adding body to your sauce." He's right and I've been doing that ever since.

Suggested reading: Simple Italian Food (Clarkson Potter, 1998).

You're Gonna Make What?

With a good recipe, the right ingredients, and the proper tools, you can cook just about anything. Think of it as the ultimate arts and crafts project that you get to eat when you're done. Virginia Willis, who is a great cook, super party caterer, and producer of "Home Plate," a cooking show on TV's Turner South, even makes fresh ginger ale for guests! Somehow it's not surprising that in Virginia's former life she was in charge of Martha's Test Kitchen for that amazingly perfect TV series . . . yes, *the* Martha! "I also use the same technique with young sassafras root to make fresh root beer and it is yummy. Sort of Laura Ingalls Wilder foraging in the woods combined with my dear gal Martha kind of a recipe. It was inspired by a shoot I did with Chef Patrick O'Connell at The Inn at Little Washington, Little Washington, Virginia." Who knew you could make ginger ale? Let Virginia's kitchen coaching inspire you to try all kinds of from-scratch recipes.

Homemade Ginger Ale

Virginia Willis, great cook and television producer, Atlanta

YIELD: *4–6 servings*

1 cup sugar

1 cup water

One 2-inch piece ginger, thinly cut into coins

Seltzer water

1. In a saucepan, bring the sugar, water, and ginger to a boil. Stirring occasionally, cook until the sugar is completely dissolved.

2. Remove from the heat and let cool completely. (Syrup may be made 1 week ahead and chilled, covered.)

3. Spoon 2 tablespoons of ginger syrup into a tall glass filled with ice. Top off with seltzer and stir to combine.

Hip & Healthy Heroine: Janet Trefethen

"Beware the Bottomless Wineglass!"

Petite and pretty Janet Trefethen, owner of Trefethen Vineyards, one of the oldest wineries in the Napa Valley, famous for gorgeous Chardonnays and classy Cabernets, who fetes and is feted a lot in her very social line of work, has this red flag for dinner party guests. "At some parties enthusiastic hosts want to make sure your wineglass stays full, so they dutifully keep refilling the glass. Then you totally lose track of how much you are drinking. It still looks like one glass, but every time you take a few sips it gets filled up again. So, heaven only knows how many glasses you really drank." When she's hosting, Janet prefers to pour a glass of wine to match each dinner course so that the quality of the culinary experience is prioritized. You should always ask the guest if they'd like more before reloading their goblet. Otherwise they'll never know when to say "when." **Carolyn Says:** The vodka version of this almost happened to me during a beautiful dinner at the Yusupov Palace in St. Petersburg, Russia. (This was the place where the murder attempts on Rasputin took place, so I should have been at least a little wary.) Seated next to vodka veteran Don Kendall, the founder of Pepsico (and legendary businessman who made the deal with the then-Soviets to get Pepsi into Eastern Europe by agreeing to market Stolichnaya vodka in the United States), I learned that if you finish the small glass of vodka before you, a waiter quickly fills it up again. Wanting to respect local traditions, but not noticing how many times my vodka kept being refilled, I enthusiastically toasted, "*Nostrovia!*" to the beauty of the historic palace, the charm of my dinner partners, and the welcoming energy of this new Russia. Was it a great night? *Da.* Would I down that much Russian vodka again? *Nyet!*

Food and Wine Pairings

First of all, know that the rules on food and wine pairing were meant to be broken! If you want Chianti with your crab cakes or Chardonnay with your Châteaubriand, that's okay. But it is fun to taste and compare different wines with food because some matches do seem to be made in heaven. It's either because they contrast wonderfully—such as a fruity Reisling with spicy Thai food—or they mesh effortlessly—such as succulent roast lamb with a smooth Pinot Noir. Janet Trefethen even pairs wines with the seasons. "It depends on the time of year, how hot or cold it is. In winter if I'm making a robust venison stew and the fire is crackling, I serve a heavier red wine such as Cabernet Sauvignon. In summer if we're doing pork tenderloin on the grill, I think Cabernet Franc goes best because of its peppery kick." BTW: You won't necessarily find it on European wine bottles, but most American and Australian winemakers put pairing notes right on their labels today. They want you to enjoy your time with food and wine!

Gourmet Guru: Hilary White

The Amazing Morphing Menu

There's no need to brainstorm entirely different menus each time you entertain. If you master a few simple recipes and techniques, you can adapt your "specialties" to the season and the occasion. Gourmet Guru and executive chef of 103 West in Atlanta, Hilary White (who at size six is another Hip & Healthy Heroine!), came up with a dream team of dishes that morph to fit your party's mood. "I've come up with a template menu, but changed the way the dishes are served depending on the party theme. If it's a fancy dinner, then do plated courses. If it's summer, start on the patio and just do a buffet. Offer dishes family-style for holiday meals." And Hilary has worked her menu magic using Dish Diva favorites, plenty of vegetables, a lean meat, and a fruit-based dessert.

So, here are the players:

- ✳ seasonal salad or vegetable
- ✳ beef tenderloin
- ✳ fruit crisp

All you have to do now is match your fashions with the festivities! Recipes for making beef tenderloin and a fruit crisp follow. Hilary shares her delicious ideas for making each meal a special occasion.

Elegant Dinner Party

Maine Lobster with Warm Fennel Salad

Roasted Tenderloin of Beef with Wild Mushrooms

Rhubarb Crisp with Strawberry Sorbet

The idea behind this is that it's plated and the guests are seated. All the food can be cooked in advance. Take into account you don't want to have to wash dishes between courses, so have your china set and ready and all silver and glassware preset. A party like this can seem overwhelming because of the high-end ingredients and because your guests are seated. Perhaps keep your guest list small to create the special occasion.

Summer Casual

Crispy Goat Cheese with Shaved Fennel

Roasted Tenderloin of Beef with Sweet Corn Relish

Peach Crisp with Whipped Cream

This variation of the menu would be great for a casual summertime gathering of friends. It's an upgrade from the typical Fourth of July or Memorial Day menus. The style of service offers platters of food, giving guests the freedom to make their own plates and join each other at tables. Slice the tenderloin in small, almost bite-sized pieces to make it simpler for guests to eat. The Sweet Corn Relish can be a mixture of what the summer has to offer: cucumber, tomatoes, corn, and a dice of jalapeños. Toss the relish with salt, pepper, vinegar, and a bit of oil and allow it to marinate to create a juice for the meat. The addition of arugula at the base of the platter would make it a meal in itself.

Holidays with Family

Roasted Tenderloin of Beef

Fennel and Potato Gratin

Cranberry-Apple Crisp

This menu is for family and friends gathering at the same table passing platters and casserole-style dishes around the table. Items can be prepared and cooked in advance to allow you to join your guests. Items of your preference, glazed carrots or Brussels sprouts with bacon, could be added to round out the menu.

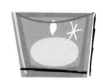

Roasted Tenderloin of Beef

Hilary White, Executive Chef, 103 West, Atlanta

Chef Note: A 5-pound tenderloin yields about 10 servings

1. Season the tenderloin with salt and pepper.

2. Place in a hot roasting pan with olive oil and sear all sides till dark golden brown

3. Remove the tenderloin from the pan and place it on a rack and back into the par

4. Roast the tenderloin at 325 degrees F until the meat reaches the internal temperature of 125 degrees F for medium-rare.

5. Remove the tenderloin from the oven and allow it to rest. Slice and garnish as desired.

Fruit Crisp

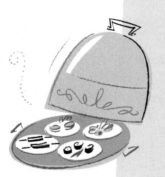

YIELD: *12 servings*

For the Topping:

1 cup oats

1 cup brown sugar

1 cup Bisquick

½ pound unsalted butter

1 teaspoon cinnamon

For the Fruit:

10 cups of fruit, cut into bite-size pieces

½ cup sugar

Juice of one lemon

1. Place all the topping ingredients in a mixer with a paddle and combine.

2. Mix the fruit, sugar, and lemon juice.

3. Place the fruit in a baking dish and cover the fruit with the topping.

4. Bake at 325 degrees F until the fruit bubbles and the topping is golden brown.

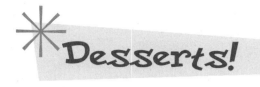

Desserts!

Your friends will be amazed. All along they thought you were the romaine lettuce–loving babe of the bunch, and here you are plating up dreamy slices of cherry torte and key lime pie. What's the world coming to? It's dessert, baby! The Dish Divas know that even if every tooth in your mouth is a sweet one, you don't have to live life without ice cream, chocolate cake, pecan pie, or even strawberry cheesecake. The sweet taste of dessert is one of life's greatest pleasures. Thank goodness food companies are just as excited about dessert and have churned out of their test kitchens low-fat frozen yogurt, no-fat fruit sorbets, low-calorie chocolate puddings, and even bite-sized cheesecake bars that control the portion for you. Of course, any time the ingredients cream, sugar, and butter enter recipe territory there's reason to slow down to calorie-caution speed. Add succulent fresh fruit to desserts and you can step on the accelerator, again knowing that you're not only enjoying sweet delights, you're getting some good nutrition and fiber in every bite too.

To Dessert or Not to Dessert?

Even if you've sworn off desserts, don't assume your guests will want to follow suit. Besides, no one, including you, should have to go dessert-free. Thinking of offering one decadent, gotta-have-it dessert and one health-conscious one? Forget it. Chances are, most of your guests will opt for the healthy dessert, whether they want it or not. (Appearances, you know.) May we suggest ever-so-small precut servings of the sweet stuff topped with a generous helping of fresh fruit or fresh fruit puree? Or find a good source for fresh fruit gelato with just a drizzle of chocolate syrup. If it's the good stuff, it tastes loads more decadent than it really is. Another option: Check out chapter 8, The Dish on Cheating, for a great ever-so-slightly modified cheesecake recipe to die for. And the sky's the limit for fresh fruit cheesecake toppings. If you really want to wow your guests with a sweet treat, try this recipe, which passes the taste test in Tinseltown! Sherry Yard, executive pastry chef at Spago, Beverly Hills, creates desserts that have to impress everyone from I've-seen-everything movie moguls to uber-slim actresses who say, "Oh, maybe just one small bite!" BTW: If we were casting Sherry in a Hollywood hit, she'd play the pixie-cute, energetic girl next door, who just happens to be one of the best dessert chefs in the nation. Sweet!

Suggested reading: The Secrets of Baking, Sherry Yard (Houghton Mifflin, 2003).

Banana Chocolate Chip Soufflé

Sherry Yard, Executive Pastry Chef, Spago, Beverly Hills

Chef Note: This is a perfect use for leftover brown (yes, super-brown and ugly) bananas!

YIELD: *10 servings in ½-cup soufflé cups*

1 cup banana "schmutz" base

8 egg whites

⅛ teaspoon cream of tartar

½ cup granulated sugar

¼ cup chocolate chips

1 Make the banana "schmutz" base (see page 265).

2 Preheat oven to 400 degrees F. Butter and sugar the soufflé cups.

3 Whip the egg whites, cream of tartar, and sugar until stiff peaks form.

4 Fold in the banana "schmutz" base and chocolate chips.

5 Pour the batter into ten buttered and sugared individual soufflé cups.

6 Bake at 400 degrees F for 13 to 15 minutes; the centers should be creamy.

7 Serve with whipped cream.

Banana "Schmutz" Base

YIELD: *1 generous cup*

8 ounces very ripe bananas	¼ cup light brown sugar
½ stick butter (2 ounces)	2 tablespoons Myers's dark rum
⅓ cup granulated sugar	1 tablespoon lemon juice

1 Peel the bananas and remove any strings and butts. Roughly chop.

2 In a large, heavy pot, heat the butter over high heat, until browned. Add the granulated sugar and brown sugar, stirring constantly, until it is a dark caramel color.

3 Add the chopped bananas and cook for 3 to 4 minutes until the bananas have broken down.

4 Remove from the heat and add the rum. Stir to combine.

5 Place back on the heat and continue to cook, stirring constantly, until all of the liquid is gone.

6 Remove from the heat and stir in the lemon juice. Puree immediately in a blender or food processor. Set aside until ready to use and allow to cool to room temperature.

Fruit Finesse

Just don't have the time to whip something up for your little get-together? Editor in chief of *Bon Appétit* magazine, Barbara Fairchild, says for dessert in a pinch, a lovely big bowl of the freshest fruit in season, with some excellent store-bought cookies and brownies is absolutely fine. From farm-stand fresh apple pies to a mix of multicolored berries dotted with crème—fruit-based desserts are definitely back; just flip through the pages of major food magazines such as *Bon Appétit*. Another dessert idea: small, delicate servings of great-quality ice cream topped with a simple fruit compote (homemade or store-bought) and sugar cookies. Serve in pretty, balloon wineglasses. Check out *www.bonappetit.com* for a treasure trove of recipes and entertaining tips.

Let's Turn the Tables

Okay, let's say *you're* the invited one. Don your festive party rags and get ready to have a good time. It's easy to be the guest, right? Smile, mingle, and say what a grand time you had as you leave. Well, there are a few more etiquette items you might want to keep in mind, if you're an invited guest who happens to be on a diet.

1 *Eat something!* Maybe everything looks fried or processed and just the overall opposite of healthy. But that doesn't mean you have to be a party pooper. Somebody went to a lot of trouble to put together that menu, unhealthy though it may be. Suck it up for one night and try a bit of this and a bit of that. Unless you've got a true life-threatening allergy to say, seafood or peanuts, there's just got to be something you can eat. You're not a food critic. For now, just enjoy the company.

2 *Don't talk diet.* Once the ball gets rolling, it's like a twelve-step program with everyone listing a litany of sins, followed by their newfound healthy eating plans. Besides, diet talk can be more incendiary than talking sex or politics. You might make the host feel guilty for not offering your special diet foods.

3 *Don't BYOF.* To show your appreciation that someone else has done the cooking, bring your host a food gift. How about an aged balsamic vinegar or extra-virgin olive oil in a beautiful bottle? Or a basket of perfect peaches or other fruit in peak season? You're spreading the good news that healthy foods are beautiful. (And not that you would, oh fashionable one, but do not *BYOF.* That stands for bring your own food. Maybe you prefer sea salt on your veggies or your own special brand of salad dressing. Save it for next time, when you're the host.)

Hip & Healthy Heroine: Claudia Fleming

"Dessert and the Dancer"

As the award-winning pastry chef at Gramercy Tavern restaurant in New York City, Claudia Fleming not only surprised guests with her culinary creativity, she often shocked them when they saw that this devotee of desserts was ballerina slim. Sure enough, she started out as a ballerina, classically trained from age eight. After a professional career in modern dance during her early twenties, she moved into another kind of show business—the restaurant world! Claudia says looking back, it doesn't seem like a weird transition. "The whole idea of using techniques, practicing, repetition of skills, and then preparing for show time—whether it's cooking or dancing—it's all very much team work and individual expression." And the results of her expression through desserts earned her top culinary awards and many happy food fans. What we love about Claudia is her dessert philosophy. "I have always enjoyed presenting small servings of several different sweets. A tiny blueberry tart, a small crème brûlée topped with raspberries, a spoon of fresh pear gelato, and a morsel of chocolate torte. It just seems like more fun to have a variety of dessert flavors and if they are really good, you don't need that much." Now that makes us want to dance!

Suggested reading: The Last Course—The Desserts of Gramercy Tavern (Random House, 2001).

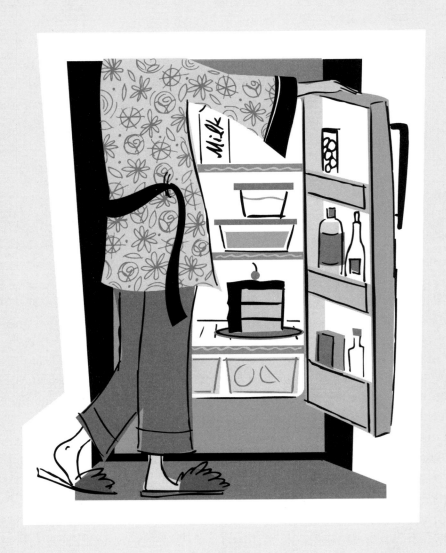

8 The Dish on Cheating

Everything in moderation, even excess!

Surprise! Cheating, falling off the wagon, losing your willpower, splurging, whatever you want to call it, can be part of a healthy lifestyle—if you know how to get back on track before you career out of control. We all deserve to indulge ourselves every once in a while! But lifelong weight-control success depends on how you define "cheating." Dietary indulgences come in a huge variety of shapes, sizes, and flavors. The worse thing to do when dipping into the cookie jar at midnight is to say to yourself, "Well, I'm really off my diet *now*, so I may as well just go for it and eat as many as I want!" Instead, take note that you really want a cookie, *now!* Eat one or two and enjoy those chocolate chips (with low-fat milk!). So, you can savor your delicious dalliance and return to your tried-and-true eating style the next day, without ever missing a beat. No harm, no foul. So, there's no need to give yourself a time-out for bad behavior. In fact, congratulations are in order every

> *Excess on occasion is exhilarating; it keeps moderation from acquiring the deadening effect of a habit.*
> —W. Somerset Maugham

time you do go a little overboard and then adjust to stay shipshape. Having said all that, we would have to be a little daft to say that there aren't occasions that make it all too easy to go off the dietary deep end, never to return. So we're going to let you in on some key triggers for out-of-control eating and share our own little "cheat sheet" that we've put together for you.

The Cheat Is On

If you're like most of us, you'll likely discover sooner or later, that cravings (sometimes triggered by emotions) are what often make you overeat, not an out-of-control appetite. Uncover the triggers that make you overeat, learn how to manage them, and you've won half the weight-loss battle already. But it's important to learn coping techniques you can live with. Because, chances are, if it doesn't feel good you won't stick with it over the long haul.

> Never eat more than you can lift.
> —Miss Piggy

Once you accept the fact that no one, and we mean *no one*, eats only healthy food 100 percent of the time, you're off the hook. No regrets, no remorse, no punishment. Just have the knowledge that, though it was yummy, you can't indulge in large portions of such decadent foods on a regular basis. Well, you can, but with your decision to indulge, you'll have to accept your cellulitic fate. And if you were ready for that, you wouldn't be reading this book, now, would you? So, read on.

She's Gotta Have It!

Think you'll just go crazy if you don't find that piece of chocolate you just know is in the bottom of your purse? Don't worry, you're not nuts. And by all means, go ahead and eat it! (Remember: It's best to savor a small serving of really good dark chocolate than slurp down a huge chocolate milk shake!) Food cravings are real and they're really pretty common, especially in women. The *Journal of Nutrition* reviewed the power of cravings and found that there are quite a few reasons they occur. While cravings can range from pretzels to pickles, the most common are for sweet foods and fatty foods, especially chocolate. And get this—don't try and trick your taste buds; a report in the *Journal of the American Dietetic Association* found that chocolate cravings are not satisfied by other sweets. Some folks have argued that cravings erupt when our body cries out for needed nutrients. Chocolate is a decent source of the mineral magnesium, so could a diet low in magnesium be causing those midnight moves to bake brownies? Could be, but spinach is even higher in magnesium. Don't often see anyone ripping open a bag of spinach to quench a craving, do you?

It's All in Your Mind

Yes, and your mind is a strong force! Some research shows that cravings for sweets (which are carbohydrates) may kick off a chain reaction increasing brain chemicals called neurotransmitters that influence mood. So, if you're feeling down, that craving for cookies might help boost your spirits. But eat too many and you'll boost your body size—that's really depressing. And if you use certain foods too often as your go-to comfort foods, you might actually condition yourself to crave them in the future. P.S. Don't forget that a little exercise can put you in a better mood too.

Conquering Cravings

Though there is research suggesting that some cravings may have a biological origin, most cravings are brought on by tough-to-rein-in emotions or out-of-control situations. Here are a few of the most common emotional triggers and tips for taking control.

Emotional Eating

Anger. If *anger* (especially suppressed anger) sends you shrieking and running for cover in the comfort of your kitchen, then you're managing your anger by eating (read overeating). While food may seem like your most dependable source of comfort, it ultimately leaves you more out-of-sorts than before. It may sound like psychobabble, but experts insist it's true. If you face the source of your anger head on, it's less likely to blow up and take control of your appetite.

Anxiety. Whatever your source of *anxiety*—an upcoming job interview, conflict at home, or an unannounced visit from your in-laws—it's a common trigger for overeating. Ask yourself, do you reach for a chocolate-filled croissant every time your mother calls? Do you pack away the sour cream and onion potato chips every time you balance your checkbook? You can't eliminate these triggers from your life, but you can try to minimize your anxiety level. First, make sure you get enough sleep. The threshold for anxiety is lower when you're not rested. Try different methods of relaxation techniques, like deep breathing, yoga, reading, listening to soft music—whatever works for you. Found a friend who enjoys doing checkbook math? Well, that works too.

Boredom. There's nothing like good old-fashioned *boredom* to bring on the munchies. Before you decide to busy yourself by ferreting through the freezer for ice cream, do whatever it takes to shift the focus away from food. Take a shower, paint your nails, throw out old newspapers or take one last look through that magazine before you toss it. Make a list of your favorite diversions and keep them posted on the fridge.

Depression. Being down in the dumps and a little *depressed* can certainly do your diet in. The occasional blue mood can take hold, now and then, and prevent you from doing the things you want to do and sometimes makes you do things you'd rather not—like overeat. Instead of letting that blue funk trigger calorie overload, view it as a call to action. Getting active is one of the best ways for lifting a black cloud. Go for a walk, a run, a bike ride, jump on the treadmill. Once the clouds have parted, you can see more clearly whether now is the time to indulge or not. Not only have you lifted your mental fog, but you've burned some extra calories. Sweet!

Happiness. Yes, it's true. Even *happiness* can make you fat. Who doesn't feel like celebrating when something good happens? A new job, a new house, a new man in your life, an exotic vacation—all make you want to celebrate, and celebrations usually involve food. That doesn't mean you shouldn't ever kick up your heels because you might overeat. It does mean that you should let common sense be your guide and learn to compensate for occasional indulgences. Overeat at a celebratory dinner—cut back the next day.

Create-a-Craving

One of the prime suspects in creating uncontrollable cravings is the well-meaning practice of eliminating certain splurge foods such as ice cream or other goodies. The lure of the forbidden fruit, you know.

✳ Wait out the Craving Storm

If you find yourself giving in to your cravings just once too often, then maybe you should try to wait them out. Psychologists have found that most cravings have pretty predictable patterns. They begin slowly, gradually gain intensity, reach a peak, and whether or not you give in, they fade away and return to normal. What should you do? Wait out the storm. If you can stop yourself from giving in, the craving will eventually fade away on its own.

Another way to create a craving is skipping meals so that your blood sugar plummets and your willpower gives in to less-than-nutritious choices. Eating higher-fiber carbohydrate foods during meals, such as oatmeal for breakfast and fruits and vegetables at lunch (especially legumes, like beans), can help keep your blood sugar off the roller coaster and your hand out of the cookie jar.

Not everyone feels food cravings but we Dish Divas know they are *real* and should be *respected*. So accept your cravings and learn how to control them, even if it does mean buying the best brand of chocolate you can find!

The Most Common Cravings

Not only do men and women differ in the frequency of their cravings, they also each have their own unique objects of their craving desires. Women tend to crave—you guessed it—chocolate, along with other sweets like cookies and ice cream. Men, on the other hand, tend to crave things like pizza and steak. But that's neither here nor there. Extra calories are extra calories that can provide extra padding on a woman's derriere or put an extra layer on a man's love handles. Remember what we said about portion control? (You can check out chapter 2, The Dish on Diet Basics, to refresh your memory.) Well, if you decide to give in to that craving, try to at least keep an eye on your portion. Giving in to that irresistible craving for white chocolate truffles is okay—but try to limit it to one and savor the taste—s-l-o-w-l-y. One is enough to satisfy that craving. Any more than that and you're asking for truffle trouble in the form of unwanted pounds.

> Vegetables are a must on a diet. I suggest carrot cake, zucchini bread, and pumpkin pie.
> —Garfield

Dear Diary

One of the best ways to identify your cravings and eating triggers is to keep a food journal. Keep a running record of not only what you eat each day, but what happened and how you felt before and after eating. Journaling is considered one of the most powerful tools for changing behavior, from anger management to weight management! You'll be surprised at what you'll uncover about your own hidden food triggers. No need to let it be an open book. It's nobody's business but yours. Continue after you've started making healthful changes in your eating habits and marvel at the progress you've made. But don't let it become an obsession. Just know that once you stop journaling, it's not a bad idea to pick it up again occasionally, for a spot check to see how you're still doing. "Dear Diary . . . can't wait to tell you what I had for dinner at Philippe's Bistro last night. And you won't believe who was there!"

Know What You're Getting Into

If you're going to splurge, it's really important to know what you're getting into. How many calories are in those fudge brownies? (250) Or that medium-size triple-thick vanilla shake? (750) Is the ice cream sundae really worth it? (As much as 1,270 calories.) How many are lurking in an order of grande nachos slathered with hot chili and melted cheese? (1,300) Okay, and how many laps do you have to swim to burn that many calories? Strap your goggles on for the long haul. The secret to splurging is picking what you want, but knowing when to stop before you've gone too far. For instance, there are just 100 calories in five Hershey's Kisses. So gobble away. And sometimes a lighter version of a treat will satisfy a craving, if you pick the right brand or the best recipe. Did you know that one cup of strawberries adorned with a tablespoon of fat-free hot fudge sauce is another 100-calorie "splurge"?

✳ Funky, Fabulous Food Facts

You've probably heard of late that chocolate has redeemed itself by virtue of the fact that it contains natural compounds, called phytonutrients, that can improve your health. So far, so good. Maybe craving chocolate is a good thing? But before you dive into that box of Godiva, get a grip! (You didn't think it was going to be that easy, did you?) First of all, you can forget milk chocolate. Only dark chocolate has the good stuff. And, second, the reasons chocolate developed such a bad reputation in the first place still remain; right along with its recently discovered health-promoting phytonutrients, all chocolate still contains the same old fat and calories.

Want a taste of the rich stuff without doing time for the crime? Try strawberries or dried apricots dipped in dark chocolate. Heaven!

Anatomy of a Cheesecake

As we've said, "The more you know, the more you can eat" and the "know" part is really important here. That way you will be able to keep track of how far you wandered off track and then cut back on calories when the cravings subside or ramp up your physical activity the next day. That's the *balance* part of the nutrition theme song—"Moderation, Variety, and Balance." Cheesecake can be the ultimate sin, rich in fat and calories, because the really great ones are made with lots of cream cheese and eggs. Some add sour cream and chocolate and just about all have a crumb crust rich in butter and sugar. Checking the nutrition stats on a full-boat, full-fat cheesecake, you can count 457 calories and 34 grams of fat per slice (one-twelfth of a 9-inch cake). Say, "Cheese!" Or better yet, say, "Jeez!!!!"

That doesn't mean cheesecake is evil, it just means you either have to split that piece with four friends or figure out a way to lighten it up without comprising its smooth and creamy, rich and cheesy, lovely allure. And that's a mission Jill Melton has been on and emerged victorious. "Even when coming up with a facsimile of a splurge food, it's always flavor first." In making their cheesecakes, the test kitchen at *Cooking Light* discovered a combination of low-fat sour cream, fat-free cream cheese, and one-third-less-fat cream cheese did the job. Fewer eggs are used in the cake and a lot less butter in the graham cracker crust. "So many cheesecakes have gobs of butter in the crust and it's just not necessary." So, cut the fat where you can, but leave it where it counts.

This recipe for Banana Split Cheesecake is just one of *Cooking Light* magazine's cheesecake creations. Go to *www.cookinglight.com* for many more.

Banana Split Cheesecake

From the miracle makers who love great-tasting healthy foods at *Cooking Light* magazine

YIELD: *16 servings*

Crust:

1 cup packaged chocolate cookie crumbs

2 tablespoons sugar

1 tablespoon butter or stick margarine, melted

Cooking spray

Filling:

Three 8-ounce blocks fat-free cream cheese, softened

One 8-ounce block one-third-less-fat cream cheese, softened

One 8-ounce carton low-fat sour cream

1½ cups sugar

1½ cups mashed ripe banana

3 tablespoons all-purpose flour

2 teaspoons vanilla extract

4 large eggs

Toppings:

⅓ cup canned crushed pineapple in juice, drained

⅓ cup strawberry sundae syrup

⅓ cup chocolate syrup

¼ cup chopped pecans or almonds

16 maraschino cherries, drained

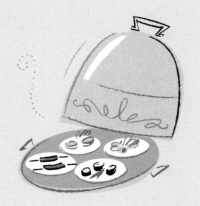

1. Preheat the oven to 325 degrees F. Coat the bottom of a 9-inch spring-form pan with cooking spray.

2. To prepare the crust, combine the first three ingredients in a bowl; toss with a fork until moist. Press into the bottom of the pan.

3. To prepare the filling, beat the cheeses and sour cream on high speed with a mixer until smooth. Add 1½ cups sugar, the banana, flour, and vanilla; beat well. Add the eggs, one at a time; beat well after each addition.

4. Pour the cheese mixture into the prepared pan; bake in the preheated oven for 1 hour and 10 minutes or until almost set. The cheesecake is done when the center barely moves when the pan is touched.

5. Remove the cheesecake from the oven; run a knife around the outside edge. Cool the cheesecake to room temperature. Cover and chill at least 8 hours. Top each serving with 1 teaspoon pineapple, 1 teaspoon strawberry syrup, 1 teaspoon chocolate syrup, ¾ teaspoon nuts, and 1 cherry.

To Snack, to Graze, Perchance to Eat?

Are you a snacker, a grazer, a three-meals-a-dayer? If you fall into the three-meals-a-day category, surveys say that you're part of a shrinking minority. It seems that snacks and meals have become interchangeable and that as a group, Americans have shifted from the typical three-meal-a-day pattern to one of constant grazing. So, where do the snacks end and meals begin? Therein lies the biggest problem. If you're always in grab-and-go mode, then it's tough to tell where you left off, both calorie- and nutrient-wise. The calories just keep piling up with no time or meal barriers to eating. Some of the most popular snack foods (chips, cookies, and snack bars) can tack on extra fat and calories before you can say, "Yum!" According to a recent survey, fresh fruits and vegetables are popular snack foods too, but it's doubtful that anyone would overdo on produce. When you're snacking, job number one is to be on "portion patrol." Take care of the portions, and the calories take care of themselves.

Snacking Secrets

It's only 10 A.M. and you're starving! You tell yourself you'll just nibble on a little something to tide you over until lunchtime, when you plan on eating less to make up for your midday munchies. Well, here's a news flash for ya. According to David Levitsky, Ph.D., the sultan of snacking research from Cornell University, you're likely to eat the same amount at meals whether or not you snack in between. Translation? If you're not careful, that snack is likely to end up being a calorie add-on, not a calorie advance toward your lunch or dinner. Don't get the wrong message. We're not saying that all snacking is bad. Just be aware that if you don't make allowances for those insidious in-between meal calories, you could end up packing on extra pounds on the sly.

Does Your Body Know What You Need?

There's a school of thought that when you crave certain foods, it's your body's way of telling you that you need more of some component of that food. You crave salty potato chips, your body needs more salt. You crave a juicy steak, you need more protein. Hard candy? You need more carbs. But is that really what's behind your secret food desires? We checked in with Adam Drewnowski, Ph.D., director of the Center for Public Health Nutrition at the University of Washington, and a longtime researcher on cravings, and posed that question. He didn't beat around the bush. "It's nonsense," he says. "The body doesn't crave what it needs." In fact, he says, the body tends to crave the things it doesn't need, like foods that are high in fat, sugar, or salt. Reach for a food that provides two out of three, and faster than you can say Krispy Kreme, you have the magic formula for a craving.

Hip & Healthy Heroine: Barbara Albright, M.S., R.D.

It's All in Your Jeans

Ever wonder what a chocolate-loving dietitian does to cope with her cravings? Well, Barbara Albright not only embraced her love of the dark sweet stuff, she dove into a full-time chocolate job as the editor in chief of *Chocolatier* magazine. Now Barb is a cookbook author and has over twenty titles to her credit, including *Margaritas, Girl Food* (with cartoonist Cathy Guisewite), and *The Garfield Cookbook* (Andrews & McMeel). "I start each and every day with just a little bit of chocolate. Usually followed by some of the orange juice my children did not finish. Then I go work out. At about ten-thirty, I eat a hearty sandwich or wrap. Later I drink a glass of wine while I make a well-balanced and hopefully interesting family-friendly dinner. I don't eat dessert and I don't usually eat late at night." (That's right, Barb . . . you *start* the day with dessert!)

Barb reveals that she does weigh herself every morning. At five eight she shares that she likes to stay between 135 and 139. "If the scale says 140 I go into panic mode and curtail my eating. Also I regularly wear jeans because they can be very telling of the state of your body; when they are tight, they act like an appetite suppressant." One more tip from Barb: Take up a hobby that busies your hands. She loves to knit and is working on two knitting books now. "I found that knitting also curtails hand-to-mouth activity. The yarn gets messy when you are eating chocolate at the same time!"

* Wild, Wild Weekends

Everyone likes to let loose and have fun on the weekends. The same goes for let's-get-the-party-started eating and drinking. And what might seem like a no-brainer has actually been confirmed by researchers at the University of North Carolina. The findings? We let down our guard and eat more calories on the weekends. How much? Here's what they found: On average, we eat about 115 calories more on Saturdays and Sundays than we do Monday through Friday. To be honest, we're surprised the calorie surplus isn't more. All that partying, munching, and unscheduled nibbling, not to mention Sunday brunch! Okay, so 115 calories might not sound like much, but over the course of a single year, the calorie grand total is equal to almost four more pounds on your hips and thighs! Your choices are two: Eat less or exercise more. May we suggest a combination of the two? And there's usually more free time to get in that workout or that game of tennis with friends. So, what are you doing next weekend?

Is It the Real Thing?

. . . .

What exactly is that sudden burning desire for warm-from-the-oven chocolate chip cookies? Is it hunger or is it appetite? What's the diff, you say? Here's the dish: If you're truly hungry, you'll feel stomach pangs and rumblings, along with that familiar gnawing feeling in the pit of your stomach. If you're *really* hungry, you may even feel a headache coming on. Appetite, on the other hand, is not your body begging for more food, it's a desire for food based on emotions, habits, moods, sights, smells, and memories. If you've had years of experience of mixing up the two, then have patience, my dear. It will take time to begin to identify which one is taking hold and sending you to the fridge in search of food.

One approach is to find your own personal hunger barometer. (**Densie Says:** Mine happens to be an apple. It has to be a healthy food that you ordinarily like.) If you think you're hungry, and your personal hunger barometer sounds *delish,* then Bingo! It's hunger you're feeling. If, however, you find yourself snubbing your barometer in favor of a dish of cookies 'n cream ice cream or a cheese danish, then you weren't hungry at all. It was your appetite that was rearing its ugly little head.

Sweet-Tooth Truth

Carolyn Says: There's a metal sculpture in Philadelphia of a shapely nose and big lips and, no, it's not calling attention to a building full of supermodels! Dedicated to the study of taste and smell, the Monell Chemical Senses Center is home to researchers who specialize in flavor and aroma research. Director of the Center, Dr. Gary Beauchamp, knows a lot about the illusive and all-powerful sweet tooth. While it's no surprise that a liking for sweets is universal, "It looks like some humans do taste things sweeter than others." A real breakthrough—Gary says genetic research today can identify genes that control sweet receptors in the mouth. "We're in the Golden Age of taste research. We've learned more about what happens on the tongue in the last thirty-six months than in the past thirty-six years!" So, in the spirit of "You can't fool Mother Nature," if you've got a sweet tooth with 'tude, don't ignore it! Choose small portions of sweet treats and see if it calms the call for confections.

Dish Divas' Cheat Sheet

Here are a few little cheating tidbits that you may find helpful in your quest to keep overindulgences to a minimum.

* *Banish guilt.* Nothing is forbidden. Once you've established that ground rule, guilt goes out the door.

* *"Cheat" in a public place.* It's no longer a clandestine meeting between you and that chocolate éclair. It's out in the open. It takes away a bit of the allure and, with it, some of the temptation.

* *Disconnect cheating from a loss of willpower.* You may have "cheated," but don't think of it as a lost battle of wills: you against food. Think of it as a decision you made. You weighed your options and decided to go for it. Now move on.

* *Aim for progress, not perfection.* You used to indulge every day, now it's just on the weekends. That's progress, but it's not perfection. Anyway, we think perfection is way overrated.

* *The more you know, the more you can (ch)eat.* We've said all along that "the more you know, the more you can eat." Well, the same rules apply to cheating on some of your favorite foods. The secret to successful cheating? Portion control. You know what we're talking about. One cookie won't do you in, but a dozen would be a serious setback. A child-sized portion of ice cream lets you indulge in your passion, without racking up too many calories. A double scoop with whipped cream and nuts, while not the end of healthy eating as we know it, does call for a little damage control.

* **To Each Her Own**

  So, it all makes sense now. That new guy at the office may make your best friend weak in the knees, but he leaves you cold. No chemistry. It's the same thing with food. A dish that makes you drool at the very thought may make someone else gag. The difference in taste may indeed be a matter of chemistry . . . genetic chemistry. Learn your own, perhaps inherited, craving weaknesses and learn to deal with them. They may be as much a part of you as the color of your eyes—treat them with respect, but don't let them dictate your diet.

* *Demystify food.* It's that love/hate relationship thing that causes all the problems. Take away some of the mystique you've built up around those "forbidden foods" and they're not so seductive anymore.

* *If you're not hungry, don't eat.* Okay, this one gets a big "duh!" But think about it. How many times have you reached for food

when your stomach was doing just fine?—thank you very much. This one requires a little internal reality check, but once you become tuned in to when you're really feeling hungry, mindless munching on favorite "cheat" foods fades into the background.

✳ Cheaters Anonymous

You're not alone in your efforts to make overindulgence a thing of the past. But you say support groups aren't your thing. Too much public confession and self-flagellation for your taste. You prefer a little privacy and confidentiality, if you please. Okay. There's this great invention called the Internet you might want to check out. Along with auction websites, booksellers' websites, and more sites to buy supplements than you can shake a stick at, come a handful of helpful diet support websites. And believe it or don't, there's actually solid research out of Brown University and Baylor College of Medicine that shows online support can make weight loss easier. Go online for e-mail, real-time, or bulletin board support, even keep online food journals to help you keep track of what you're putting in your mouth. Studies show that all this Internet interaction can help dieters lose up to three times more weight that those who go it alone. And part of that success comes from getting online support to ride the wave of cravings with someone to "talk you down."

Some of the sites are free, while others charge a fee of about $15 to $20 a month. Here's a sampling of some sites you might want to give a shot to help you cope with your food issues.

www.WeightWatchers.com   *www.caloriescount.com*
www.eDiets.com   *www.e-nutrisystem.com*
www.ivillage.com

So who said cheaters never win??? Now that you know the rules of the games, so to speak, you get to enjoy the foods your crave, and keep everyone wondering, "How *does* she do it?"

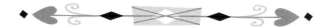

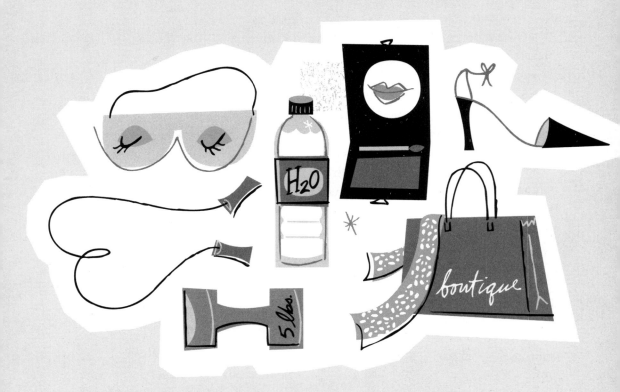

9 The Dish on Looking Fabulous

"**Wow! You really look great!**" are five of the most powerful make-you-smile words in any language. It's good to know that whatever you're doing to slim down, rev up, and feel good in your clothes, and in your own skin, is not only working for you—it's noticeable to your friends. Positive feedback is a great motivator to keep on doing what you're doing. What's new? Maybe it's a long overdue haircut or you're wearing a color that gives your skin a healthy glow. Or maybe you were inspired during your last aerobics class when the instructor told everyone, "Don't underestimate the power of posture! You'll look five pounds thinner if you remember to stand up straight." In this chapter, we want to give you the lowdown on high-energy fitness and share some of the best tips of the health and beauty trade. First, let's get moving!

> You can't change where you came from. You can change where you are going.
> —Anonymous

The Dish on Getting Active

As you'll soon learn, you can't talk diet without talking exercise. Slimming down by calorie-cutting alone is just too tough! So, we're going to give you the dish about how other stylish women get active and stay active. From our dietitian friend who "rewards" herself with 5 A.M. junkets to the gym, to our frequent traveler friend who, while at a hotel, will stay only on the same floor as the exercise room, we'll share the "been there, done that" from smart women. We'll give the naked truth about the best ways to burn calories. Go on, get jiggy with it! Break into some drop-butt dancing in the middle of the room with the music at glass-shattering volume (clothing optional). Not only will you burn calories, you'll instantly feel edgier, sexier, and more vibrant. Maybe spinning, kickboxing, or Pilates is more your style. We'll give you some pointers to help you find the physical activity that's right for you.

"No Pain, No Gain"— Oh Yeah? Says Who?

Do you really need to "feel the burn" to benefit from exercise? Just how much is enough? Well, that depends on what you're after. If you simply want to look and feel better and burn off some extra calories while you're at it, then you don't need to push yourself to the outer limits of your endurance. If you're planning for the next Boston Marathon, then there will definitely be pain involved. The truth is, any physical activity on a regular basis is good for your health, your weight, and your self-confidence. Experts say, for the record, that exercise is a must-have for managing your weight. Diet alone just won't cut it. Undeniable, real-life proof of that comes from something called the National Weight Control Registry, a national database of successful losers, who have taken off an average of sixty-seven pounds and kept it off for at least five years. It's not a diet program. Each one of the four thousand people in the registry does his or her own thing and reports back to the record keepers. The revealing truth is that 89 percent of the success stories changed not only their diets, but their physical activity as well.

The Official Word on Exercise

Okay, so we've established that you probably don't need to run marathons to feel better and lose a few pounds. But just how much exercise should you set your sights on? Is two hours a day too much, twenty minutes not enough? It really depends on whom you ask. Serious fitness buffs, who measure body fat and live from one workout to the next, might give you a different answer from experts who are interested simply in getting you up off the sofa.

Here's the dish: The experts at the Centers for Disease Control and Prevention in Atlanta and the American College of Sports Medicine, both organizations worth listening to, recommend at least thirty minutes of "moderate-intensity" physical activity (swimming, walking briskly) at least five days a week. The Institute of Medicine, however, recommends twenty or more minutes of "vigorous-intensity" physical activity (bicycling uphill, jogging) at least three days a week. It's sort of six of one, or half a dozen of the other, if you ask us, but there you have it. Research shows either one can benefit your health. But you can't ignore the advice from those who have "been there, done that" from the National Weight Control Registry, who say they exercise sixty to ninety minutes a day to manage their weight. Anyway, one-formula-fits-all approaches just don't work in real life. The best approach? See what works for you. If you're trying to whittle away five to fifteen pounds, maybe you don't need ninety minutes a day. Check with your doc, start off slowly, and see where it takes you. We like the "five-minute factor" approach. Start off with fifteen minutes of walking, jogging, biking, hiking, whatever. Then after you've done that for a while—a few days, a few weeks—and get comfortable with it (you suddenly realize you're no longer huffing and puffing when you're done), then add another five minutes. Keep it up until you've reached your own magic number for managing your weight.

Time vs. Intensity

To burn an equal number of calories, the formula is simply higher intensity = less time; lower intensity = more time. Here are a few exercise categories to choose from, courtesy of the folks at the CDC and the American Council for Fitness and Nutrition.

Light-Intensity Activities

* Walking slowly

* Golf, powered cart

* Swimming, slow treading

* Gardening or pruning

* Bicycling, very light effort

* Dusting or vacuuming

* Conditioning exercise, light stretching or warm-up

Moderate-Intensity Activities

* Walking briskly
* Golf, pulling or carrying clubs
* Swimming, recreational
* Mowing lawn, power motor
* Tennis, doubles
* Bicycling five to nine mph, level terrain, or with a few hills
* Scrubbing floors or washing windows
* Weight lifting, Nautilus machines or free weights

Vigorous-Intensity Activities

* Racewalking, jogging, or running
* Swimming laps
* Mowing lawn, hand mower
* Tennis, singles
* Bicycling more than ten mph, or on steep uphill terrain
* Moving or pushing furniture

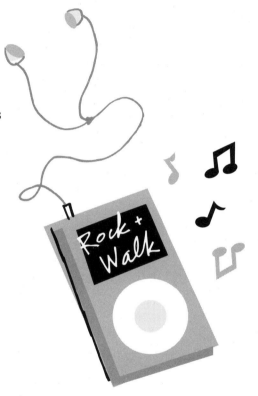

Weight vs. Time

Your current numbers on the bathroom scale figure into the calorie-burning formula, right along with exercise intensity. Curious about how many calories you're burning? Check out these 100-calorie burners.

(These calorie-burning numbers apply if you weigh 130 pounds. If you weigh less, you'll have to hang in there longer to burn off 100 calories; if you weigh more, you'll burn the calories faster . . . you get the idea.)

EXERCISE	MINUTES
Jogging	10
Jumping rope	10
Swimming	12
Rollerblading	15
Biking	16
Aerobics	17
Ice skating	17
Yoga	19
Walking briskly	18
Walking the dog	23
Cleaning house	29

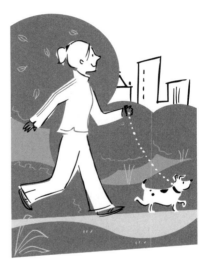

Power Shopping as Exercise

The calorie-burning potential of this one has yet to be determined by CDC researchers, but it only makes sense that you'll burn a few. You're a woman on a mission, trekking from store to store, looking for just the right shoes to go with that amazing new outfit. But your total calorie burn depends on how long it takes you to find those shoes, how far you have to walk (is it the Mall of America or the local strip shopping center?), how far you park (how about parking a little farther away from the storefront, rather than searching for the closest spot you can?), and how many shopping bags you're schlepping around. The more you carry, the more calories you burn. But, hey, let's not forget to deduct those calories consumed in the Food Court. You could end up calling it even.

Just Get Off Your Derriere, and Move!

Those sweaty Nike commercials have been urging us for some time now to "Just Do It!" But according to a recent survey, most of us are not heeding the call to perspire. The survey done by the Centers for Disease Control and Prevention in Atlanta found that more than half of all adults don't get the recommended minimum amount of activity. Which half do you want to be in?

Carolyn Says: I exercise for two reasons: Sanity and Vanity! When I hit the 3½-mile trail that wraps around Chastain Park in Atlanta I know that the brisk walk in winter, spring, summer, or fall will make me feel better and clear my mind. Sometimes I go with friends and talk about stuff—that's good for the soul. Sometimes I go alone and enjoy the silence—another way to beat stress. But every time I finish the loop, I know that moving my butt will keep it from moving on its own! I want to feel good and look good—sanity and vanity!

Feeling Fabulous over the Long Haul

If you see your efforts to lose weight and keep it off as a Sisyphean* task you'd rather not be saddled with forever, there's good news. Researchers quizzed over nine hundred successful losers, again those guys and gals from the National Weight Control Registry, and found that keeping the weight off got much easier with time. As the years passed, they reported less effort and attention was needed to keep their weight on track. We kid you not. How is that possible? Here's a theory: After years of successfully managing your weight, what once seemed like a burden becomes second nature. And the rewards of a healthy diet and exercise far outweigh any sacrifices (walking instead of driving, eating a sliver of cheesecake instead of a half-pound slab; having a small, single scoop of ice cream instead of double-dipping).

* In case you've long since forgotten your Greek mythology, Sisyphus was the greedy king of Corinth who was doomed in hell to roll uphill a heavy stone, which always rolled down again. Substitute a few extra pounds for the stone, and well, you get the idea.

A, B, C's of Aerobics

. . . .

When you decide to hop on the fitness bandwagon, aerobic exercise is likely the first stop. The term "aerobics" was coined in 1968 by Ken Cooper, M.D., founder and president of the Cooper Aerobics Institute in Dallas, Texas. And it stuck. (It's no coincidence he's known in fitness circles as the "father of aerobics.") If you think back to Biology 101, you may even recall that "aerobic" literally means to require oxygen. So, aerobics is exercise that needs oxygen. And it's not just conformist exercises done to disco tunes in packed gym rooms. Any activity that gets your muscles moving, gets your heart pumping, and gets you breathing faster than normal will do the trick. Think swimming, walking, jogging, martial arts, dance. One new form that sounds like fun and we think is worth a try is "rebound aerobics" done on a mini trampoline. You're a kid again, jumping up and down on your bed, but the instructor is telling you to keep it up, rather than, "cut it out, right now!"

✳ Don't Worry, Be Happy

According to John Foreyt, Ph.D., a psychologist and director of the Behavioral Research Center at Baylor College of Medicine in Houston, physical activity may raise levels of endorphins in the brain, compounds that promote a sense of well-being. If you feel good on the inside, then you look good on the outside. Any exercise will do the trick, but better make it regular.

There are even "punk rock aerobic" classes we found in Boston and New York, if that's your thing, complete with "classic" punk rock tunes. Here's a rundown of some aerobic exercises you might want to check out. Oh, and it's a good idea, no matter your age, to get the okay from your doc before you decide to go all out with exercise.

Walking Away from *Extra* Pounds

Walking is what you might call your "no-excuses" exercise. (Didn't that used to be a brand of jeans? Oh well.) The advantages are many; let me count the ways: Almost everyone can do it, it's free (except for a comfortable pair of shoes), it's almost always available (except in truly horrid weather), there's minimal risk of injury, and you can map out your own plan of action— hilly, flat, fast, slow, long, short, alone or with an exercise buddy. Of course, for true cardiovascular fitness, you'll need to kick it up a notch from a leisurely stroll to speed-walking or power-walking, but any walking at all is better for your body than sitting like a slug on the sofa. Researchers now know that regular walkers have healthier hearts, sharper minds, and less body fat. How much walking is enough? The experts have tallied up steps and say that, yes, a good ten thousand steps a day is enough to improve your physical fitness. But twelve thousand to fifteen thousand a day is more likely to help you lose weight. To put that into perspective, bear in mind that the average person takes somewhere in the paltry neighborhood of five thousand or six thousand steps a day. The only way to know how close you're coming to the goal is to count (no, you don't have to keep a mental log, silly). Invest in a pedometer. It's a little pager-size gizmo that you attach to your waist and it'll clock off every little step you take. Best source: *www.new-lifestyles.com*. You can get the basic, no-frills model or one that has memory and tells you how many calories you've burned. There's a cute, bright yellow one that says it's designed for kids, but check it out. The others come in basic black or blue.

> Walk This Way!
> —Aerosmith

Run Like the Wind!

Okay, so maybe you'll never even break the turtle-paced twelve-minute mile, but hey, if you're running, you're definitely on the right track, so to speak. Whether you're running as fast as you can or jogging along at a more leisurely pace, it's a great aerobic activity and calorie burner. But it's not for everyone. If you're starting out with more than just a few pounds to lose, running may not be the best way to start. Something a little less strenuous, at least in the beginning, would be a better approach. And for all you busty ladies out there, don't even think about it without investing in a good sports bra that offers plenty of support. If you've ever had knee or back injuries, then all that pavement pounding might not be too smart either. But if you don't have any of those things to hold you back, then go for it. Get a good pair of shoes (don't go cheap on the shoes or your feet will suffer), jogging gear appropriate for the weather, a CD player and headphones for some tunes, and you're good to go. Just be sure to stretch before you run, start off slow, and work your way up. Listen to your body. If it says it's time to rest, then obey. If you push too hard your first time out, you may not be motivated to go a second time.

Want to get into running? There are lots of women-only races these days that are designed specifically to encourage women to get physically active. (Translation: Not everyone there will be a super-fit, die-hard runner.) Check your local newspaper.

The Power of a Personal Trainer

These personal guides to physical fitness are not reserved for the rich and famous anymore. If you have the will and the way to fork over $35 to $100 an hour for a little one-on-one tête-à-tête with an expert, then by all means, give it a try. As any floundering student in school can tell you, there's nothing like individualized tutelage for shortening the learning curve and getting it right the first time. But trainers don't always carry the holy grail of exercise; certification isn't regulated by any state or federal agency. (And you're much better off going to a sports nutritionist for diet advice. Unless, of course, your trainer is qualified to do both!) Having laid those cards on the table, if you're debating whether to sign up with a personal trainer to get you on the right track, there are lots of reasons why it's a good move (it's motivating, your workouts will be more consistent and more effective, and if you've chosen the right trainer, you should get a little ego boost from the "way to go, girl" that you'll hear when you get it right). But the most important advice of all . . . find someone you feel comfortable with. If all you're looking for is a little guidance and understanding, you don't want to sign up for ten sessions with a workout dominatrix, who's going to make you run screaming from the gym to the nearest exit. Find a trainer who's right for you and then, instead of asking yourself if you can afford it, maybe you should be asking if you can afford not to?

Spinning for Fitness

In case you haven't heard, riding a stationary bike has been upgraded to "spinning." Sort of the next generation of the activity. Created in the 1980s by personal trainer and ultra-endurance athlete Johnny G, it's an indoor group-cycling program. Though its roots may be in stationary cycling, spinning is a group activity; you cycle to music and instruction, and it incorporates loads more variety than just cycling away on your own. And because of the way the classes are designed, you get much more resistance training than you would from regular cycling—at least for your legs. You'll need to work on your upper body another way. But be forewarned; spinning classes come in all levels. If you're a beginner, don't even think about signing up for an advanced class. You could spin out of control! For more info on spinning and to find a place where you can spin, check out *www.spinning.com*.

Hip & Healthy Heroine: Nicole Kerr, R.D., MPH

Are You Stairing?

It's no surprise that taking the stairs instead of riding the elevator or escalator is the right move. But did you know that it burns five times more calories? It's also considered what experts call a weight-bearing exercise, so it's good for your bones. Stairs too grungy where you work or live? Registered dietitian Nicole Kerr got her bosses to spring the funds to spruce up the stairways in her office building so more folks would feel good about the climb. They painted the walls bright colors, added carpet, fun posters, brighter lights, and even some music. But no boring elevator music here—the tunes run from disco on Mondays to wind-down classics on Fridays. Nicole's figured it out. "If you take the stairs for ten minutes a day, up and down, and you keep your diet constant in the course of a year, you could actually lose ten pounds!"

Okay. Now we'll tell you where she works—the Centers for Disease Control and Prevention's Division of Nutrition and Physical Activity in Atlanta. So, maybe it was a little easier than most to get the higher-ups to spring for the renovation. But research shows the stairs are being used a lot more often now and Nicole talks to groups all across the country about the importance of adding easy activity back into our lives. Be a Hip & Healthy Heroine at your office or apartment building—initiate a staircase makeover! Tell 'em the CDC sent you!

Jumping Rope

"Cinderella, dressed in yella, went upstairs to kiss a fella . . ." Ah, a childhood game of jump rope. If you have dewy-eyed memories of this favorite playtime activity, well, it's time for an update. Now that you're all grown up, jumping rope is no kid's game; it's a heart-pumping, muscle-building, calorie-burning, all-weather exercise that can keep you fit with minimal time and planning. In fact, jumping rope is a serious fitness business. There are even national championships that air on ESPN. Not that you feel like training for the next competition, but it can be motivating to watch. So, how to get started? There's not much too it. If you jumped rope as a kid, it's like riding a bike. You may stumble and feel like a klutz for a few minutes. But once the memory kicks in, legs, feet, and arms begin to cooperate. Start off slow; it can leave you breathless after just a minute or two if you're not used to it. Just make sure you get a rope that's long enough, so you don't trip yourself with each hop, skip, and jump. Our friends at *www.jumprope.com* offer these guidelines for choosing a jump rope that's right for you:

YOUR HEIGHT	JUMP ROPE LENGTH
Up to 4' 10"	7 ft.
4' 11"–5' 3"	8 ft.
5' 4"–5' 10"	9 ft.
5' 11" and over	10 ft.

Your Target For Being Fabulously Fit

You may have heard the hard-core gals at the gym going on and on about their target heart rates. It's the gold standard for how far you're able to push yourself, without entering the danger zone. If you're superfit, your heart and lungs may be so efficient that you never reach your so-called target; if you're totally out of shape, you may reach it with little effort and have to be careful not to go overboard. But it's a target worth aiming for. Here's how it works: First you figure your *maximal* heart rate. The formula is simple: Take 220 and subtract your age. The older you are, the lower your maximal heart rate. Your *target* heart rate is lower. When you exercise, your target heart rate should be 50 to 80 percent of your maximal heart rate. If you're new to exercise, stick to the lower end of that range. Too complicated? Here's an example: If you're thirty-five, your maximal heart rate would be 185 (220-35). If you're a beginner, your target heart rate would be 50 percent of that, or 92. As you get more fit, you can nudge your target heart rate up a bit.

Pilates, If You Please

You could say it's the yoga for the new millenium. Though it's been around for ages (some of the first people to use the Pilates Method were dancers such as Martha Graham and George Balanchine), Pilates has become the "hot" activity for fitness seekers only in recent years. It offers more resistance training than yoga, but is equally effective for stretching and building strength, without bulking you up. The method focuses on using fewer repetitions of more precise exercises that challenge the abdomen, lower back, and buttocks. When these super three muscle groups are strong, the rest of the body is able to move freely and with grace. The routines offer a series of controlled movements using specially designed exercise equipment, but you may have to go through basic mat exercise classes before you'll be allowed to use the equipment. The Pilates workout machine looks something like a cross between a rowing machine and a torture rack. But don't let that put you off. It's a great workout.

For more information on Pilates and how to get started, check out *www.pilates-studio.com.*

Karate Chop Those Pounds

We don't pretend to be martial arts experts, but lots of women find self-defense classes a great way to blow off steam, while building strength, confidence, and grace. Okay, so maybe none of us will ever be up for a role in *Matrix IV* or be ready to duke it out with Xena Warrior Princess, but this exercise really kicks butt! Literally! Whether you pick karate or kung fu, tae kwan do or tai bo, here's a primer to get you into the body-toning action. Oh, and be sure to sit on the sidelines to watch a class before you sign up. Some of them can be pretty intense. Since you're there for the fitness, not the fighting, you might want to look for classes that train you to be a hot body, not a bodyguard! Don't have a clue what's the diff between karate and kung fu? Here's a quick martial-arts primer to get you started.

Aikido—The Japanese art of unarmed self-defense. It encourages discipline and nonviolence. Movements include joint twisting, grabbing, and bending.

Get the picture: Steven Seagal uses this style.

Karate—Concentrates on kicking and punching. An offensive and defensive martial art.

Get the picture: Remember *The Karate Kid?*

Kung Fu—Used more as a generic term for martial arts, though there are many different styles that barely resemble one another.

Get the picture: Think Jackie Chan meets Xena Warrior Princess.

Jeet Kune Do—A combination of the best of many styles of martial arts.

Get the picture: Bruce Lee invented this one. 'Nuf said.

Kickboxing—Sort of a cross between karate and kung fu, blended with boxing.

Get the picture: Jean-Claude Van Damme, "the muscles from Brussels," is known for kickboxing movies.

Tae Kwon Do—A Korean martial art that involves mostly kicking.

Get the picture: Check out Jennifer Garner on the tube in "Alias."

Carolyn Says: I took a year of Shotokan karate while I was at Florida State University and although I never got beyond a yellow belt (is that for coward?), I did learn to kick backward, block a punch, and flip a tall guy. It improved my posture, tightened my desk-bound butt, and I really liked the outfit.

Whatever It Takes

No matter which activity you choose, or whenever you choose to do it, the number-one rule is to make it work for *you*. Everyone is different; so what works for your longtime gal pal won't necessarily work for you. And what worked for you ten years ago just might not be what you need today. **Densie Says:** A fellow nutritionist friend of mine likes to "reward" herself with 5 A.M. trips to the gym to work out. Somehow "reward" and "5 A.M." seem like a contradiction in terms to me. The word *masochistic* comes to mind, however. But, hey, it's worked for her for years. Another friend who travels a lot for her job always calls ahead to locate the exercise facilities in the hotel and asks for the closest available room. It's harder to ignore and talk yourself out of it, if fitness is just a few steps away. When you make it a part of who you are, rather than something you simply have to do, physical activity becomes as much a part of your life and your routine as eating, bathing, and snoozing.

✳ Water by *the* Numbers:

During exercise, drink 28 to 40 ounces of fluid per hour.

✳ Drink Up!

Okay, you're ready to work out. Just be sure you get plenty of fluid (for more on your liquid choices, check out chapter 6, The Dish on Drinks). According to a recent study done at the Gatorade Sports Science Institute (yes, there really is such a place), nearly half of all exercisers arrive at the gym already dehydrated, even though they believe they're doing just fine. And even minor dehydration affects your ability to pump that iron, kick up those legs, and spin those wheels, making your workout feel like a chore, rather than an energy booster.

Hip & Healthy Heroine: Julie Upton, MS, R.D.

Born to Run

Densie Says: I've known Julie, a sports nutritionist in New York City, for years, and she's always been enviably fit and active; she runs, she bikes, she swims. She even does Ironman triathlete events. But it wasn't until recently that I found out regular physical activity, and lots of it, has been a part of her life since she was a kid. The sports nutrition gig was a natural career choice for her. Obviously, for Julie, it's in the genes. She's got those magic muscle fibers that beg to be challenged. As a natural born fan of fitness, it would be easy to be less-than-empathetic for all us nontriathlete types. But she has some incredibly useful advice for the rest of us fitness-freak wannabes. Despite living in New York, where there's an endless supply of spas, gyms, and work-out rooms catering to every lifestyle, Julie says she hasn't been to a gym in years and still stays fit. Good news for gals on a budget. She says it's easy to do on your own. Running, walking, or biking are good, heart-healthy, calorie-burning activities you can do without belonging to a club. And, she says, resistance training to build muscle strength can be done even without working out at a sweaty gym. How so? Old-fashioned sit-ups, push-ups, squats, or wall-sits. (You back up against the wall, with your feet a few inches out and gradually slide down until you're in a sitting position. You'll definitely feel the burn.) They all use your own body weight to build and strengthen the major muscles.

Her other basic advice is to set goals, no matter how small. "I want to run a 10-minute mile, instead of a 12-minute mile." Or, "I want to run in the next local 5K race." Or, "Next year, it's the New York City Marathon!" or maybe it's more along the lines of shaping up for vacation, swimsuit season, or a really hot date. Whatever sets the fire. "I've set zillions of goals," says Julie. "I haven't reached all of them, but they've kept me motivated and given me something to look forward to."

✳ Pumping Iron, with Style

Shopping around for hand weights, but would rather avoid the stark look of all that heavy metal and chrome? Check it out. Now you can bring your keen fashion sense along for the ride while you pump iron. Pick your own palette: Be pretty in pink, start your day off with a little burst of sunshine yellow, seafoam green, or maybe bright blue? There are several shopping sites online that offer these soft, comfortably padded hand weights, ranging from one to ten pounds each. For starters, try: *www.bodytrends.com.*

Get a Body Buddy
. . . .

So, who's your body buddy? Friends are one of the most powerful forces in helping you keep your promise to work on fitness goals. Researchers at the University of Pittsburgh and the University of Minnesota's School of Public Health became "study buddies" and proved that friends who followed a weight-loss program together lost more weight and were more likely to complete their diet program and maintain their weight loss than those who did it alone. And in a recent Weight Watchers survey, one-quarter of the women polled said that they met their weight-loss goals because of help from a friend, who acted as a motivating coach: "Yes, we will do our bike ride today!" or provides a comforting ear: "Don't worry, we are going to do it together!"

Healthy Cell Phone Plan
. . . .

Your exercise buddy doesn't even have to be in the same city. Need a friend to keep you company walking around the park? Why not take your cell phone and talk while you walk in Peoria and she walks in Portland?

Whether your walking shoes take you through the mall, around the park, or through the neighborhood, you can use this time to return your mom's phone call or catch up with an old friend. It's the ultimate in multitasking. You're burning calories while you're yakking. Maybe this will help your motivation: If you can add ten minutes of walking on the weekdays at a moderate three mph pace, you'll burn about a thousand calories a month and lose three pounds a year—the healthiest way to use your cell phone minutes!

Hip & Healthy Heroine: Jane Fonda

Sleek and Serious Role Model

Carolyn Says: The first time I saw Jane Fonda in person she was drinking bottled water at an Atlanta Hawks' basketball game. She was sitting in the front row next to team owner Ted Turner—her then-husband and my then-boss. As everyone around her guzzled beer and gobbled sports night snacks, she cheered on the team, happily hydrating with H_2O. I thought, I know they say to drink plenty of water to keep your skin and body healthy. She's taking that advice seriously. I think I'll get some bottled water too.

The next time I saw Jane, we were at a CNN ten-year anniversary party and she enthusiastically said hello and then sprang into action. "Ted! This is Carolyn. She does Nutrition for you on CNN! Isn't that great?" Wow! Thanks, Jane. BTW: She always looks great. Whether it's a black-tie gala or a ballgame, she is glamorous. Great hair and makeup are the keys, but I think it's her carriage that counts most. She glides into a room, standing tall but relaxed. As an actress she was trained to communicate with language and body language, lessons learned from just watching Jane Fonda. Then there's the lesson learned from listening to Jane. As founder of the Georgia Campaign for Adolescent Pregnancy Prevention (G-CAPP), she speaks about the significance of teaching girls about the strength of inner beauty that comes from promoting a powerful sense of self-esteem. Whether you're a teen or a baby boomer with big plans for the rest of your life, Jane Fonda is a fabulous role model for every girl.

Looking Good Just Standing There

Remember when your mother/grandmother/aunt/second-grade teacher/ballet instructor (insert additional well-meaning, bossy type) told you to "Stop slumping and stand up straight!"?

They were offering you one of the least talked about but best pieces of fitness advice going—the importance of good posture. It's even part of the "improve your body, mind, and soul" fitness philosophy at Canyon Ranch Health Resort in Arizona where Dr. Michael Hewitt, Research Director for Exercise Science, says with your shoulders pulled back, chest out, and stomach in, "You look more fit and appear taller." Hey, instant weight loss! And because so many folks spend their days hunched over a computer keyboard or a steering wheel, the muscles responsible for good posture can actually get lazy. "Many women I see have rounded shoulders. It's actually uncomfortable for them to pull their shoulders back. It's not a strength issue. It's muscle memory." To improve your posture, he says you can train the muscles in the upper back and chest to make good posture effortless. He suggests exercises where you are pulling, like the action on a rowing machine. Strong abdominal muscles help support the back too. Another posture plus, "Good posture is important while you're working out. You'll target the right muscles and it can help prevent fatigue and injury." Are you sitting up straight?

✳ Klutz Control

There's more to physical fitness than just burning calories and pumping iron, says Dr. Michael Hewitt of Canyon Ranch Health Resort. Physical activity, whether it's dance or tai chi, bull riding or ice hockey (hey, whatever floats your boat), will help you become more agile and graceful, two traits that give you that *je ne sais quoi*—a total boost to your fabulous factor.

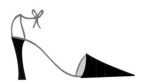

Burning Calories Just Sitting There

Muscle power helps you carry that overpacked suitcase down the stairs and lift a case of bottled water out of a grocery cart. And you've heard it before, "Use it or lose it!" That's definitely true here. Canyon Ranch's exercise guru Michael Hewitt says beware of "sarcopenia." No, it's not an exotic muscle-eating microbe, it's the scientific name for muscle weakening from lack of use. "By the age of thirty or thirty-five women lose six to seven pounds of muscle mass and it's simply replaced with flab." To make matters worse, when what was muscle disappears and is replaced with fat, your metabolism slows down so you burn fewer calories. To rev things up again you have to increase lean body mass by pumping a little iron. "Dieting and aerobic exercise such as walking can help you reduce body fat, but you have to do some strength training to increase lean tissue." (Michael suggests using light weights and doing many repetitions until the muscles feel fatigued.) Here's the big payoff. When you become leaner and your muscles are stronger you'll actually burn more calories, even when you're just lounging around, compared to when you were marshmallow soft. We're not talking muscle beach, iron-pumping bulk. This is the kind of muscle tone you want to see in sleek legs and firm arms. But a word to the wise: Since muscle weighs more than fat, don't freak if you actually weigh a little more. Michael explains, "The numbers on the scale are meaningless. You could be a few pounds heavier and a dress size smaller because lean mass is more dense." Hey, Skycap! I'll carry my own suitcase!

Fidget Away Fat

There's another little-known way in which you burn calories by just sitting there . . . well, sort of. It's called NEAT, and it stands for "nonexercise activity thermogenesis." Translation? Nervous bodies in constant motion, even if it's not exercise, require more energy. When you bounce your leg under the table, stretch while sitting at your desk, rock back in forth in your chair, or tap your fingers on the table, you're fidgeting away calories. Don't laugh! We're serious. Researchers have studied it and found that the fidget factor can actually explain the differences in weight gain among some people. For those Nervous Nellies who can't seem to truly sit still and relax, all that unnecessary movement can actually burn enough calories to prevent them from gaining weight.

Retro-Fit

They may not have gone to yoga, sought out fat-free frozen desserts, or counted fat grams on a Palm Pilot. But poodle-skirted women of the 1950s were able to eat less and exercise more than today's designer active-wear generation. Research done by editors at a British woman's magazine, *Prima,* found that the housework and other activities of daily life in 1953 (think walking to the market, hanging out the laundry, only one family car, no TV) burned up more than a thousand calories a day. Compare that to the average woman today, who burns half that much and consumes more calories—2,178 a day now, as opposed to 1,818 then. Why the calorie climb? There weren't any fast-food places or much junk food in the fifties and the study suggested that women in 1953 were more likely to cook meals from scratch and include fresh vegetables. *Prima* editor Maire Fahey reflects, "It is telling that modern technology has made us two-thirds less active than we were. It goes to show you the importance of exercise in the battle to maintain a healthy balance."

Hip & Healthy Heroine:
Mary Ann Browning

Advice from the Fittest of the Fit

She was a graceful, reed-thin, principal dancer with a South African dance company for eight and a half years who experienced eating disorders and bad health before turning to exercise and physical fitness as a way to get healthy again. She credits a fantastic trainer for changing her life for the better. Now, Mary Ann Browning is a certified fitness trainer herself, a sports nutritionist and a triathlete, with a sculpted body to show for it, but most of all she's a tirelessly enthusiastic advocate for getting women to be as fit as they can possibly be. A specialist trainer at David Barton Gym on the Upper East Side of Manhattan, she counsels the rich and famous of NYC, but she has rock solid advice for the rest of us as well. And, she says, she practices what she preaches. Here are some of her top tips:

1. *Mix it up.* Don't get stuck on running or spinning or Pilates, or any single activity. Your muscles become more efficient with time (translation: they burn fewer calories) and you'll need to introduce new activities and alternate your routine during the week.

2. *Weight train.* She says it's incredibly important for women to build muscle and strength, without "bulking up," so make strength training a regular part of your get-fit-and-stay-fit program.

3. *Exercise five days a week.* It may seem like a lot to squeeze into your busy schedule, but she says it's the best way to get fit.

4. *Develop a personalized routine.* What works for your exercise buddy may not work for you. A good personal trainer should individualize your fitness program as well as your goals.

5. *Gradually increase your skill level.* Don't jump into an advanced Pilates class without mastering the first level. "That's like telling someone to perform *Swan Lake* when they can't even execute a plié properly." You're asking for trouble.

6. *Love yourself!* Mary Ann says, "If a woman can look in the mirror and like what she sees, then I've done my job."

You Look Fabulous!

Dress to Look Like Less

"Do these jeans make me look fat?" A good friend will tell you the truth—*before* you leave the house! And if the answer truly is, "No, they don't!" then congratulations! You've found a style that's best for you *and* you've got a running buddy who's a keeper! When it comes to choosing the right thing to wear to help you look your best, maybe those know-it-all fashionistas don't really know it all. Who invented cargo pants anyway? Don't you love how the huge side pockets sit right on the outer thighs and make you look like you've got saddlebags even when you don't? We're not suggesting a retro wave back to caftans, but there are a few fashion rules to shop by if you want to look slimmer and trimmer. (BTW: We did notice that the hipline is clean in the latest cargo pants and the cool pocket accents are nearer the knee. Could this be consumer demand in action?)

One of our favorite websites for fashion advice is *www.dressingwell.com*. We scrolled around and distilled a few tips from editor Mary Lou Andre to help you strategically minimize, using your wardrobe.

1 *Aloha!* Large prints and plaids and patterns tend to make you look larger. So the opposite applies. Small patterns in fabrics and tinier textures in knits make the areas they cover seem smaller.

2 *De-pleated.* Pleated pants can make you look wider at the waist. Opt for flat-front pants instead; they help smooth out your profile. Ditto on pleated skirts that add extra "flare" to hips you'd rather hide.

Hip & Healthy Heroine: Betsy Crawford

Personal Best

Carolyn Says: The best personal shoppers know when to state the fashion facts, and Betsy Crawford won't hesitate to tell you, "Take that off, it's not for you!" As a wardrobe consultant for the Worth Collection in Atlanta, she works with women in her home to find just the right look and the right fit—and her customers come in all shapes and sizes. "A consultant's goal is to make each client look and feel wonderful in garments. This can be achieved by using the cut of garments and certain fabrics in different ways. For instance, the extremely tall customer will always want to use some horizontal lines in clothing because it will minimize her height." Betsy believes a great belt is a tall girl's best friend. But if your goal is to try and look more like that tall gal, then think "interior and exterior column dressing." That's when the interior column of your outfit is all one color. For example, an espresso brown sweater is worn over espresso brown suede pants. "Then you can add an exterior column in a contrasting color. A below the hip length red jacket, let's say." This way, you're elongating the line of the body through color.

Betsy's Big Three

1   Use color as an accessory—accentuate your face with a scarf or your bustline with a brilliant blouse. People do have a comfort level with their favorite colors.

2   Believe that alterations are a way of life to have the perfect fit. Size matters, but if the hips are just right and the waist is too big—get the garment altered to fit you!

3   Invest in good foundation garments—they're essential to have clothes look their best. There's more to consider than just panty lines.

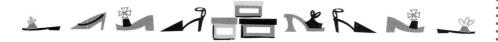

3   *Think in one color.* Monochromatic matches in one color from top to bottom will automatically make you look slimmer and taller. It doesn't have to be black.

4   *Don't cut yourself in half.* Dark on top and light on the bottom can make you look shorter and wider. Who wants that? If you're wearing khakis, pair them with a shirt in a lighter color that's flattering to your face to draw the eye up.

5   *Go ahead, have a fit!* Fit is critical because clothes that are too tight or too big won't flatter your figure. Oversized clothes from T-shirts to tuxedo pants will make you look and feel bigger than you are. Baggy clothes often accentuate flaws.

6   *Tempted to tuck?* Don't be. If you're short-waisted or working on whittling your waist, untuck your tops to lengthen your torso and appear sleeker through the middle. Avoid elastic bottoms, shirttails (too sloppy), and knit tops that are too long.

7   *"V" is for very sexy.* A V-neck is more flattering than a crew neck because it makes you appear taller and leaner and certainly makes your neck seem longer. How low should you go? Flaunt 'em, if you got 'em, girls.

8   *The Beltway.* It's always a good idea to match your belt to your pants or skirt color. If you wear a red belt with white pants it may be very nautical but it screams, "Hey, sailor! Look at my waistline!" Great if you've got a Britney Spears midriff. Otherwise, skip it. Oversized belt buckles are a bad choice too, unless you want to look like the Heavyweight Champion of the World.

9   *Skirt chasers.* A pencil skirt that reaches just above the knee is very slimming. Always the fashion choice of Alfred Hitchcock's glamorous leading ladies. They got Cary Grant, didn't they?

10 *Put that back in your locker!* Oversized T-shirts and painted-on stirrup pants can make you look like a watermelon on toothpicks. You gotta look good while you're working on looking good. Bootleg-cut gym pants balance out your hip and tummy area and are just hipper than legging-style pants. Looser-fitting running pants with the zippers at the ankles are a good choice too. We like the ones with the contrasting racing stripes down the side. You look fast and fit. And in the multitasking modern world, you can run a few errands in style on your way home.

Drugstore Beauty

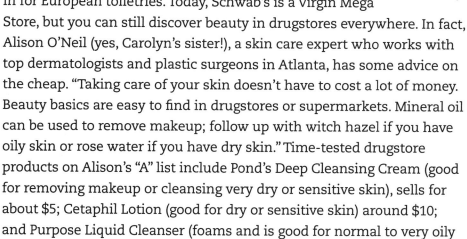

Hollywood legend has it that movie star Lana Turner was discovered sitting at the soda counter of Schwab's Drugstore on Sunset Boulevard. More Schwab's celebrity sightings—Ava Gardner shopped for face cream and Brigitte Bardot stopped in for European toiletries. Today, Schwab's is a Virgin Mega Store, but you can still discover beauty in drugstores everywhere. In fact, Alison O'Neil (yes, Carolyn's sister!), a skin care expert who works with top dermatologists and plastic surgeons in Atlanta, has some advice on the cheap. "Taking care of your skin doesn't have to cost a lot of money. Beauty basics are easy to find in drugstores or supermarkets. Mineral oil can be used to remove makeup; follow up with witch hazel if you have oily skin or rose water if you have dry skin." Time-tested drugstore products on Alison's "A" list include Pond's Deep Cleansing Cream (good for removing makeup or cleansing very dry or sensitive skin), sells for about $5; Cetaphil Lotion (good for dry or sensitive skin) around $10; and Purpose Liquid Cleanser (foams and is good for normal to very oily skin) about $7.

Alison also loves those all-in-one cleansing cloths sold in drugstores and supermarkets now. "They're terrific for after exercise, for during travel or for the occasional late night out when you're just too tired to do the whole facial cleansing routine." One more cheap trick from Alison: "Got a blemish? A spot of toothpaste (antibacterial qualities) left on overnight will help calm and clear a spot for an important meeting the next day."

Feed Your Face

Your skin wants you to eat a healthy diet too. Many nutrients, including protein, vitamins, minerals, oils, and water affect your skin's health. Nutrition may even play a role in keeping you looking younger because skin cells need certain nutrients to repair and regenerate. (This is also true for healthy hair and nails!)

When registered dietitian Lenore Greenstein was doing research for her weekly nutrition column for the *Naples Daily News* in Florida, she was amazed to find so many food links to skin health. "We know to use our sunscreen in Naples even when we're not going to the beach, but I wanted my readers to know how their diets could affect skin health." Here's what she found:

Vitamin C is essential for the formation of collagen, which is a spongy network of fibers that keeps skin plump and wrinkle-free. Good sources of vitamin C include citrus fruits, red peppers, dark green leafy vegetables, tomatoes, strawberries, and kiwifruit. The mineral *zinc* is involved in wound healing and the formation of new collagen. It is especially important for those people who suffer from acne. Good food sources of zinc include oysters, legumes or beans, nuts and seeds, oatmeal, poultry, wheat bran, and wheat germ.

Antioxidants are substances that protect against the oxidation or breaking down of cells in the body, including the skin. Many foods are rich sources of antioxidants, which protect collagen from damage by the free radicals that destroy cells.

The best protection is an array of antioxidants, from brightly colored fruits and vegetables. Try to include dark green leafy vegetables, broccoli, blueberries, cantaloupe, pink grapefruit, red peppers, carrots, sweet potatoes, squash, plums, purple grapes, beets, and tomatoes in your daily dietary plan. Don't want to look like a prune? Eat more of them. Prunes, also called dried plums, are superhigh in protective antioxidants.

There's something to that "fountain of youth." Drinking *water* throughout the day keeps skin moist and helps rid the body of toxins. Overdoing it at the bars or even coffee bars can show on your face too. Avoid excess alcohol and caffeine, which can dry and dehydrate your skin, robbing the cells of needed water, and causing fine lines to be more visible.

Protein is also essential for cell repair. Good sources of protein include poultry, fish, lean meat, eggs, low-fat dairy products, soy foods, legumes or beans, nuts, seeds and nut butters, such as peanut butter or almond butter.

Healthy fats such as monounsaturated oils help keep skin moisturized from the inside out. Healthy fats are necessary to absorb fat-soluble vitamins A, D, E, and K. Many monounsaturated fats also contain vitamin E, which is a powerful antioxidant. Lenore says, "I am always worried about fat-phobic people. They don't realize dry skin and thinning hair can be a side effect of a diet that's too low in fat."

Good sources of "moisturizing" monounsaturated fats include extra-virgin olive oil, grape seed oil, avocados, raw or dry-roasted nuts, seeds and their natural nut "butters." It's omega-3 fats to the rescue again—this time promoting healthy skin. They can be found in seafood such as salmon, trout, sardines, tuna, and sea bass, as well as ground flaxseeds, Brazil nuts, walnuts, and pumpkin seeds.

What About Food on My Face?

Cucumber slices to sooth puffy eyes. Fruit facials. Milk baths. Foods have been sought-after ingredients in beauty treatments for centuries. Genevieve Monsma, deputy beauty editor at *Marie Claire* magazine, notes, "Cleopatra used a lot of stuff from the kitchen. She may not have known it, but it was the natural lactic acid that softened her skin as she bathed in milk." So, there is something to this marriage of science and beauty! Genevieve says women today are very tuned in to "natural" products whether it's in their grocery carts or their mascara. But that doesn't mean natural-sounding "foodie" ingredients make a product better. Don't be fooled by avocado creams, chocolate body wraps, or brown sugar scrubs. Genevieve warns, "Some smell great and are even edible and they may sound luxurious to the mind, but not really be any better for the body. Just be aware that you are being marketed to."

✳ A Little Pampering Goes a Long Way

Okay, so it has nothing to do with nutrition or physical activity, but it sure makes you feel good. And that positive feeling carries over to other areas of your life, like your commitment to a healthy diet and exercise. We're talking about massages, facials, rubs, scrubs, peels, manicures, and pedicures, whether at a spa, a hair salon, or the dermatologist's office. How many other opportunities do you get to sit back, relax, and let someone else pamper you from head to toe? Come on now. How does it make you feel? Fawned over, more attractive, and in control? Go ahead, harness that I'm-worth-it feeling and use it as a motivator to eat the healthiest foods you can find and get moving.

> Don't underestimate the power of pampering.
> —Dish Divas

What's New, What's True

Green Tea Glamour

Beauty news alert for all you glamour girls: Exciting new research out of the Medical College of Georgia suggests that an antioxidant compound (EGCG) found naturally in green tea may actually help skin cells rejuvenate. Here's the dish on how green tea might work: Your skin cells are constantly renewing themselves—out with the old, in with the new. As cells come to the surface of your skin, they pretty much hang around waiting to die. And as you age, that turnover rate slows, leaving your skin looking less than fresh and glowing. What the researchers found was that the green tea compound actually brought those dying cells back to life. Energized skin cells mean healthier-looking skin. But before you drop everything and run out to buy truckloads of face cream laced with green tea, there are a few important "yes, buts" to this story. The research was done on skin cells in the lab, not on real, live faces. And it was done with concentrated amounts of only one compound found in green tea. Most skin care products that contain green tea have only small amounts or they contain a combination of all the antioxidant tea compounds, not just EGCG. But the findings are definitely something worth following.

Until the final word is in, look for products with the most concentrated amounts of green tea or green tea polyphenols (the chemical name for all kinds of antioxidants in tea) you can find. Or, you can whip up a do-it-yourself green tea treatment. Try equal amounts of brewed green tea (cooled, of course) mixed with almond flour for a natural facial scrub. Or mix brewed green tea with rice flour for a soothing green tea mask. No guarantees, of course, but it can't hurt and it might just wake up those skin cells and get them glowing again.

Spa Living Is *the* Life for Me

You've been thinking about splurging and going to a spa to whip yourself into shape. But admit it, you're a little intimidated by the whole upscale, chi-chi, superbods-on-parade thing. If so, you're missing out on a real opportunity to recharge your batteries and get a new lease on your healthy lifestyle. Not all spas are heavy on the intimidation factor. A case in point: Nestled near Lake Austin, away from almost everything else in Austin, Texas, is the Lake Austin Spa Resort. (**Densie Says:** Since it's just a hop, skip, and jump from my Austin digs, I decided to check it out. And, I'm soooo glad I did.)

While the spa is not cheap, and it's been visited by such celebs as Sandra Bullock, Jennifer Aniston, and Andie MacDowell, it's definitely laid back, much like Austin itself. And it's got a colorful history. It has been a fishing camp, a boot-camp-like fat farm, even a nudist colony. But that was then; this is now. It's located in a beautiful rustic setting on the lake, complete with all the usual spa trimmings, plus it's warm and inviting. The recently completed twenty-five-thousand-square-foot spa area, where you can get pampered to your heart's content, either solo or with your significant other, offers everything from green tea therapy to a sea salt body polish. You can get exfoliated, massaged, waxed, wrapped, or peeled. But they take their clients seriously and also offer nutrition-counseling services by a dietitian, to help you stay on track once you leave, and a certified fitness trainer to design an exercise program that's right for you.

For more information on the tons of spas across the country, go to *www.spafinder.com*. We think it's the best single source around.

✳ You Glow, Girl!

Healthy skin is number one on your list of glamour girl must-haves. Here are some top tips for taking care of your skin, keeping it healthy, and postponing those signs of aging for as long as you possibly can.

1. *Don't forget your sunscreen.* At least an SPF 15. They're not as greasy as they used to be, so they are easier to use every day. *Cosmetic caution:* Some foundations include sunscreen, but not the kind to block out harmful UV rays—so they're not a sunscreen replacement.

2. *Exfoliate.* Scrub-a-dub-dub to get rid of tired old skin cells and let the new cells glow. Skin care experts prefer physical scrubs for body such as granular cleansers, loofah sponges, or other bath scrubs. For facial skin, which is more sensitive, they suggest a chemical exfoliator such as those containing alpha hydroxy acids or fruit acids. *Cosmetic caution:* Always follow with moisturizer to protect new skin and don't over-exfoliate, which can actually damage the skin and even cause drying and wrinkling!

3. *Cleanse and moisturize.* This is where it gets really personal. Work with a skin care expert to find the right products for you, depending on your skin type, and then remember to use them! And always remember to remove your makeup and apply moisturizer before you go to bed. You're not only getting needed rest, your skin is hydrating to look refreshed the next day too. *Cosmetic caution:* If you dip your fingers into the face cream jar over and over you can actually contaminate it with bacteria. Make sure your hands are clean or use creams that come in a pump container.

4. *Exercise.* Based more on intuition and word of mouth than science, we highly recommend regular exercise as a way to give your skin that glamour girl glow. What can physical activity do for

your complexion? It gets your heart pumping and your blood flowing to all parts of your body, including your skin. You're moving your body and it shows!

P.S. If you want to find a cosmetic dermatologist near you, check out *www.aad.org*. Click on "public resources," then "dermatologist profile."

Bloat Busters

If your jeans suddenly feel too tight and you just can't suck it in, chances are it's only temporary because you're bloated. Feeling bloated is a common complaint and there's something you can do! Dr. Donnica Moore, an expert in women's health—*www.DrDonnica.com*—offered us these tips to counteract that all-too-familiar bane of female existence—fluid retention:

* Drink, drink, drink—water, that is. Though it seems counterintuitive, the more water you drink, the more fluid you'll flush out of your system.

* Grapefruit juice (six ounces per day) is also a "natural" diuretic that may help control bloating.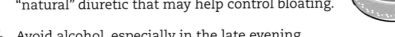

* Avoid alcohol, especially in the late evening.

* Eat fruits and veggies, as well as other high-fiber foods. These foods also "flush out your system." Carbs, on the other hand, absorb water.

* Move it! Exercise gets everything moving and can help prevent constipation, which contributes to that bloated feeling, big time.

* Get an adequate calcium intake. Studies show that women who don't get enough calcium are more likely to experience bloating. How much do you need?—1,200 milligrams a day if you're

premenopausal; 1,500 milligrams a day if you have passed menopause. For most women, that means calcium supplements are in order to get what you're not getting in your diet.

✳ Find out if you're lactose-intolerant. If you are, avoid or limit milk and other dairy products, which cause bloating. But be sure to get your calcium in supplements.

✳ Some doctors think magnesium deficiency may also contribute to bloating. The amount of magnesium contained in a multivitamin is generally enough to battle bloat. Magnesium-rich foods include artichokes, dark chocolate, dried beans, fish, oat bran, soybeans, and spinach.

✳ Control your sodium intake. Go easy on the salt-shaker in the kitchen and skip it at the table, when you can. But make a mental note that lots of prepared foods and beverages have more sodium than you might think.

"Tall and Tanned, and Young and Lovely."

Okay, you may not look exactly like the "Girl from Ipanema" who inspired the song, but you can have the tan! *Marie Claire's* Genevieve Monsma, who is naturally as fair as Gwyneth Paltrow, takes the time to use a self-tanner on her legs. "Self-tanners are so much better than they used to be and I think a tan is slimming." The ultimate treat, if you are going on a beach vacation or want to bare your arms and back in a sexy dress, is a professionally sprayed-on application. Genevieve says, "They range in price from $25 to $125. The inexpensive places are like a car wash, while the best are applied by a technician who can even customize your tan, giving you more on your legs, for instance." Add some slightly shimmery body lotion to your spray-job and you're ready for Ipanema.

Love Your Hair!

No more bad hair days! A great haircut is the link to locks that fall into place even when you feel like falling down after three sets of tennis or two sitcom's worth of treadmill time. Hair stylist to the stars (and all his other smart clients), French-born Frederic Fekkai, with salons in New York, Los Angeles, and Palm Beach, says, "My goal is to create a cut that is natural, effortless, and chic." (Imagine his French accent— "sheeeeek.") Since modern gals are on the move at the gym, through the airport, and bouncing from car pool to corporate boardrooms, there's not much time to fuss with hair that won't cooperate. Salon solution? Ronald Braso, one of Frederic's most sought after scissor sultans, believes, "Hair is the ultimate accessory, isn't it? The best styles lead to a look that fits you and it shouldn't even be noticeable that you have a cut." (Imagine his crisp British accent!)

Can the right haircut make you look thinner? Taller? More Fit? Ronald says, "Absolutely! And the wrong style can do just the opposite. It's all about proportion. If your stylist doesn't consider the shape of your face, length of your neck, and even your height, then find a new stylist!" And if you've been wondering why your hair feels dry, thin, and just won't bounce anymore, Ronald says, "Maybe it's your diet. Sure, the right hair care products (with protein and moisture) can help, but healthy hair needs to be fed from the inside too." He has seen too many clients whose dull, lifeless hair reveals their penchant for crash diets or junk food. So, feed yourself well and your hair will respond. What's the point of looking sleek and slim if you don't take care of your crowning glory?

Suggested reading: Frederic Fekkai: A Year of Syle (Clarkson Potter, 2000).

Okay, Sleeping Beauty ... Time for Bed!

We don't need a study to tell you that getting a full night's shut-eye does wonders for your complexion. Just take a good look at your skin under those bathroom bulbs the morning after you've stayed out just a wee bit too late for a night or two. It looks flat, uneven, and well, tired. No wonder it's called "beauty sleep." And the unattractive effects of doing without your nightly slumber is magnified with each passing year. The solution for this one is truly a no-brainer—get some sleep! But everyone has different sleep needs and body clocks. (**Densie Says:** Me? I'm an early-to-bed, early-to-rise kind of gal—eight hours will do nicely, thank you very much. Carolyn, on the other hand, likes to stay up late and sleep in. We both get the sleep we need, but each according to her own unique body clock.) Just do what feels right. If you wake up feeling bright-eyed and ready to take on the world, then you've gotten just the right amount of sleep for you. It's much cheaper than a cabinet full of expensive bottles of cream, lotions, and potions, and the results are guaranteed. Your complexion will thank you.

✳ You Snooze, You Lose

Anyone who believes the promise that a product can help you lose weight while you sleep must be dreaming! But as long as we're in the bedroom, let's get the real connection between shut-eye and weight control. Sleep is a must-have for your body's immune system. Obviously, the healthier you are, avoiding colds, flu, and the like, the more energy you'll have to stick to work-out goals. And a bad night's sleep adds to the nightmare of coping with life's little stresses, which can lead to overeating. Study after study reveals women turn to food to soothe themselves when it all just gets to be too much. In fact, research shows that when you're sleep-deprived, either in quality or quantity, the hormones that regulate fat cells are thrown out of whack, making weight loss even tougher. So, getting a good night's sleep not only helps you wake up looking refreshed and feeling ready to take on the world, it's actually a powerful ally in your efforts to keep those extra pounds at bay.

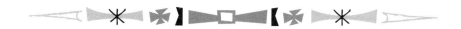

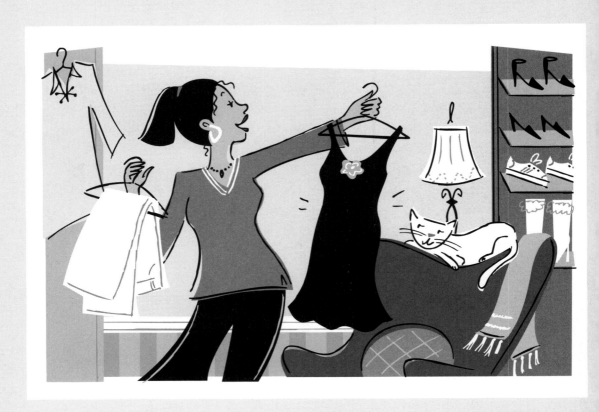

10

The Dish on What to Eat Today and Every Day (depending on the kind of day you're having)

What's a diet book without a diet plan? Well, it's true most diet books tell you what to eat every day for a few weeks, but we don't think that approach is all that helpful. What happens if we say, "Wednesday lunch: tuna fish sandwich on whole wheat with an apple," and then you get invited out to celebrate an office mate's birthday? You might think, all is lost. *Au contraire!* We're here to give you some guidance on what to eat today and every day, depending on what kind of day you're having! Remember, it's not just a way of eating; it's a way of thinking to adapt to life's little surprises.

> Life is a combination of magic and pasta.
> —Federico Fellini

In a Perfect World

To start out, we thought we'd visit the gold standard of good eating and take a look at what it means to eat right, meal by meal. To do this, we've laid out the nitty-gritty on what nutrition researchers say is best, and then we take a look at what three days of making healthy food choices looks like dish by dish, decision by decision by decision. This doesn't mean you can't stray (and eat more) and then pay (with extra activity) when you want to or need to. And since these are the habits in a perfect world, you're not to blame if you can't stick to the meal plan—because nobody's perfect. That's a relief!

Nutrition by the Numbers

According to the calculator-wielding powers that be at the Food and Nutrition Board of the National Academy of Sciences, here's what's recommended daily for healthy women to maintain good nutritional status.

At-a-Glance Daily Nutrition for Women

	WOMEN AGES 25 TO 50	WOMEN OVER 50
Calories	2,000	2,000 or less
Protein	46 g	46 g or less
Fat	65 g or less	65 g or less
Saturated Fat	20 g or less	20 g or less
Carbohydrates	304 g	304 g
	(60 percent of calories)	(60 percent of calories)
Fiber	20 g to 35 g	20 g to 35 g
Cholesterol	300 mg or less	300 mg or less
Iron	18 mg	8 mg
Sodium	2,400 mg or less	2,400 mg or less
Calcium	1,000 mg	1,200 mg
Vitamin C	60 mg	60 mg

How Does That Translate to Real Food?

Based on the architecture of the USDA Food Guide Pyramid (with a few home improvements) here's *The Dish Diva Pyramid* to help plan your dietary day.

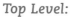

Top Level:

Fats, Oils, and Sweets: Use these to sparingly accessorize your diet.

Diva note: Choose healthy fats such as olive oil, canola oil.

Second Level:

Milk, Yogurt, Cheeses: 2–3 servings

Meats, Poultry, Fish, Eggs, Dried Beans, and Nuts: 2–3 servings

Diva note: Choose low-fat dairy, lean meats, and vegetable proteins.

Third Level:

Vegetables: 3–5 servings

Fruit: 2–4 servings

Diva note: For super nutrition, eat way more produce than this!

Bottom Level:

Bread, Cereal, Rice, and Pasta: 6–11 servings

Diva note: Choose fiber-rich whole-grain breads and cereals.

Side Dishes:

Alcohol: in moderation

Physical activity: every day

So, How Much Are You Serving Up?

Eleven servings from the bread and cereal group may sound like a silo full, and nine servings of produce may sound like a whole roadside stand, but servings are *not* that big. Maybe this will help:

Grain Serving:

* 1 slice of bread

* 1 ounce of cold cereal

* ¼ cup of cooked cereal, rice, or pasta

* 1 tortilla

* ½ bagel

Vegetable Serving:

* 1 cup of raw leafy vegetables (like lettuces or spinach)

* ½ cup of cooked vegetables (carrots, broccoli, etc.)

* ¾ cup of vegetable juice

* 1 large tomato

Fruit Serving:

* 1 medium apple, pear, orange

* ½ banana

* ½ cup cooked or canned fruit

* 17 grapes

* 1 cup cantaloupe or honeydew melon

* ¾ cup of fruit juice

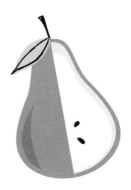

Dairy Serving:

✳ 1 cup milk or yogurt

✳ 1½ ounces of cheese

✳ 2 ounces of processed cheese

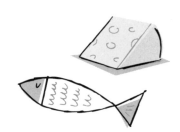

Meat and Vegetable Protein Serving:

✳ 3 ounces of cooked lean meat, poultry, or fish

✳ ½ cup cooked dry beans or 1 egg counts as 1 ounce of meat

✳ 3 ounces canned tuna

✳ 2 tablespoons of peanut butter or ⅓ cup of nuts counts as 1 ounce of meat

Fats: (Even though the Pyramid says, "use sparingly" we thought you'd appreciate a more specific definition! Each of these contain approximately 5 grams of fat and 45 calories.)

✳ 1 teaspoon of butter, margarine, or mayonnaise

✳ 1 tablespoon of reduced-fat margarine or mayonnaise

✳ 1 teaspoon of any oil

✳ 1 tablespoon of salad dressing

✳ 2 tablespoons of reduced-fat salad dressing

✳ 1 slice of bacon

✳ 1 tablespoon of cream cheese

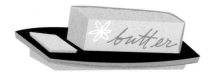

Three Days "In a Perfect World"

. . . .

Let's Try It on and See If It Fits

To illustrate how these milligrams and micronutrients might fit into the real world, we picked three days as a template for our dietary trifecta. A workday where you stay home that night, a workday that leads to dinner out on the town, and a weekend day that ends up at your place entertaining friends. We call it "in a perfect world" because we know that schedules change and willpower wanes! But based on maximizing the adage "Eat your vegetables," here's a tasty trio of fat- and calorie-controlling meal plans. (Note: These meal plans are not meant to be a diet prescription ensuring you get a specific calorie count or the perfect number of milligrams of every nutrient every day.) Good nutrition is cumulative over time. Some days are lighter than others, some days are better for calcium, some for iron. But each day of our menus should supply all of the vitamin C you need! (BTW: That's 60 milligrams of vitamin C per day.)

Thursday

Wake up! Wake up! Get out of bed! It's almost time for work and there's no time to work out this morning. But don't skip breakfast, or research shows you'll end up eating more mid-morning or at lunch. (What's that about borrowing from Peter to pay Paul?)

Breakfast

* Pop two *whole-wheat waffles* in the toaster oven for a quick and easy whole-grain breakfast.

* What are waffles without *maple syrup?* Just don't get carried away. A tablespoon or two is more than enough. Or flavor ½ cup applesauce with a little maple syrup and spoon that on top. This fruit serving adds a little fiber and a smooth contrast to the crunchy waffles.

✳ A six-ounce glass of *calcium-fortified orange juice* adds another fruit serving with a day's worth of vitamin C.

✳ *Coffee with milk and sugar.* Low-fat or skim is best, but a little whole milk is okay too if you're not using that much. Minimize the sugar, if you can.

Business Lunch

✳ *Four ounces grilled salmon* gives you those healthy omega-3's, plus more than half your protein for the day. Just remember, few restaurants dish up such small servings. Eat half (or less).

✳ *Steamed asparagus* is a great pairing with salmon, but if it comes with a heavy sauce, ask for it on the side. All you need is a drizzle of sauce to really add to the flavor. Don't forget lemons are calorie-free and are great on both the fish and the asparagus. (Bigger restaurant portions are a good thing here. One cup counts as two vegetable servings.)

✳ A small *multigrain roll* adds texture, flavor, and fiber. These are the quality carbs.

✳ *Butter*—think a *pat* of butter, not a *stick*! You're accessorizing, remember?

✳ *Seasonal berries*—restaurants usually have fresh berries. A multicolored mix adds even more nutrition. Applying the "use sparingly" strategy, enjoy a teaspoon of whipped cream on top. A great way to get fruit and dessert in one fell swoop. (BTW: one cup of berries counts as two fruit servings.)

✳ *Mineral water with lime*—no alcohol for you; you've got to be on your toes! What if your client wants to drink wine? Then enjoy a glass of white paired with your salmon and sip it slooooowly, as you take in every word!

Action Plan! Is there any way you can walk to the restaurant for lunch? Or at least pick a spot far enough away in the parking lot that you get a little walking in before and after eating? Ever notice how fit those valet parking guys are? There's a reason!

Break Time

✳ Lunch out means you'll probably have to work a bit later today. So reward yourself late afternoon with one piece of *almond biscotto.* Much lighter than a pastry, but oh, what a pairing with a steaming hot cup of joe! And the crunch is a real stress buster.

Eating In Tonight

Tonight it's just you, your TV, your fashion magazines, and your new ice-blue velour loungewear. And that's just fine with you.

✳ Grill up a *veggie burger.* (For suggestions, check out chapter 4, The Dish on Eating In.) Put it on a *whole-wheat bun* with lots of *romaine lettuce, tomatoes,* and top it off with some great *flavored mustard* and maybe a dash of *salsa.*

✳ Cook up an ear of *super sweet corn* and instead of butter, use a *reduced-fat spread* to cut calories and cholesterol.

✳ A glass of pinot noir helps elevate this veggie meal to big-time burger status.

✳ *One delicious orange,* eaten section by section as you flip the remote, helps celebrate the solitude.

Action Plan! While watching TV tonight, take the time to do those muscle-lengthening, stress-reducing stretches. Since no one's there to see you, why not do this while wearing a moisturizing face mask? It's spa night!

Late-Night Snack

✳ A glass of *skim milk* or *1 percent milk* adds to the evening's calm and gives you a calcium boost for the day. How about enjoying it with a small piece of your favorite dark chocolate? Or maybe a couple of those Thin Mint Girl Scout cookies you have stashed in the freezer? Hey, Boy Scouts! This is what *we* mean by being prepared!

It's Friday. TGIF!

You're going out for dinner with friends, so take it easy on intake during the day so you have more calories to spend on cocktails and cuisine tonight. Besides, you want to eat lean to look lean in that new red dress your man bought for you! (It's a perfect world, remember?)

Action Plan! You actually get up early enough to hit the home treadmill, or take a brisk walk for 20 minutes before jumping in the shower.

Breakfast

✳ Empty one carton of *lemon yogurt* into a bowl, add ½ cup of *blueberries*, and top it off with *honey-toasted wheat germ*. You'll love the sweet crunch the wheat germ adds and you'll be amazed at what a great nutrition package it is. (Or sprinkle on some Grape-Nuts.)

✳ A six-ounce glass of *grapefruit juice* adds another fruit serving, and since research shows that grapefruit juice can act as a natural diuretic, this is the drink to keep bloating at bay. (It's a *slinky* red dress, isn't it?)

✳ On the way to work, stop to grab a cup from your favorite coffeehouse. Steamed nonfat milk adds very few calories and a lot of fooled-ya, rich-tasting froth.

Lunch Before Your Friday Feast

✳︎ It's Food Court time or quick service at the company cafeteria. Try a grilled chicken *veggie wrap* or a big salad with grilled chicken and a small roll. Whether it's the sandwich or the salad, go easy on the dressings. Keep it simple, for tonight we dine!

✳︎ *Iced tea* with *lemon*.

Mediterranean Mod: That New Italian Place

✳︎ What happened to the antipasto?! Happily, more contemporary Italian restaurants have said *arrivederci!* to those platters of heavy meats, cheeses, and salty pickled vegetables. Instead, choose an appetizer that features *grilled vegetables* such as eggplant, zucchini, and red peppers. A few shavings of melt-in-your mouth aged Parmigiano-Reggiano cheese on top add a nutty richness. Drizzle on a little olive oil and balsamic vinegar to taste. Pair this with a glass of Pinot Grigio, a light Italian white wine that's perfect to begin a meal.

✳︎ Don't forget that real Italians eat their vegetables! Before you choose your main dish, comb the menu for interesting vegetable side dishes. You can even make it your entrée if it's a protein-rich dish such as *lentils and kale*—an often-overlooked, hearty and healthy dish.

✳︎ In the mood for pasta? *Perfecto!* This is where portion control comes into play. Do any of your friends want to split a serving? That way you both get to enjoy the carbs without the carbo loading! Order a dish like *shrimp fra diavolo*, pasta tossed with shrimp in a spicy, tomato-based sauce. (High-fat cream sauces are not for your perfect world day!) Pair this dish with a simple smooth red wine, such as an Italian Barbera.

✳︎ *Fresh lemon gelato* or *fresh orange sorbetto*. Gelato is sort of a cross between ice cream and sorbet; *sorbetto* is Italian for sorbet!

✳ *Espresso with a lemon twist.* A teeny-tiny cup of rich coffee flavor-packed with the juice you'll need to fuel that dance machine!

Action Plan! Friends say, "Let's go dancing after dinner." Burn, baby, burn, it's a calorie inferno. Dancing also helps improve your posture and your agility. Nice moves!

Saturday in the Park

Action Plan! Okay, so you slept in a little. Good for you. Sleep is nature's battery charger and you need it! But now get ready to put that healthy energy to work and celebrate Saturday with a run in the park, a hike with friends, a refreshing swim, or bike ride to the beach. Plan on getting at least an hour of intense activity today, because you've got the time!

Power Brunch

✳ Whip up a *veggie omelet.* The sky's the limit on this one. You can make it using three whole eggs, or one whole egg and two whites. Add *red pepper, green pepper, onions, mushrooms,* and *zucchini*—whatever you've got in the vegetable bin. First sauté the onions and other veggies to bring out their flavors. Set aside and then add to the almost done omelet, fold, heat through, and enjoy. A delicate sprinkle of sea salt will make these eggs sing. (See page 136, for omelet-making tips.)

✳ Cut a big *juicy tomato* in half, sprinkle the cut side with Parmesan cheese, broil, and enjoy both halves with your omelet (one vegetable serving).

✳ *Whole-wheat toast* with *whole-fruit* spread and a touch of one of our recommended *healthy bread spreads.* (See chapter 4, The Dish on Eating In.)

The Dish on What to Eat Today   335

✳ Choose your 100 percent *juice*. A growing variety of juice combos are there for the picking—orange/banana, orange/strawberry/banana, orange/passion fruit, orange/grapefruit, or orange/tangerine. Pick and pour.

✳ Brew up some *English breakfast tea* for a break from your weekday coffee habit. Hot tea will give you a lift without a full-tilt caffeine buzz. (Caffeine comparison: six ounces brewed coffee, 101 milligrams, black tea, 38 milligrams.)

Lunch on the Go

You ate breakfast a little late and you're having friends over for a cookout tonight, so you won't need a big lunch. But since today's the day you're out on your activity adventure, you should pack a healthy afternoon snack that travels well. In separate plastic bags, pack a handful of almonds, about ten baby carrots, and a sliced apple. Throw in a power bar, in case you need something more. Listen to your body's true hunger signals. To hydrate, drink some water before you head out and bring more bottled water with you too.

Dinner at Your Place

Back at home, get ready for some casual entertaining. Chill the beer and sparkling waters. Open the Merlot. How about an easy menu of *London broil* on the grill, *baked potatoes* in the oven, and a huge *tossed salad*? Your guests will have to give your salad a "10" because that's the number of ingredients in this super-tasty, super-crunchy veggie sensation. No, the inspiration for this did not come from some hippie commune. Rather, the very hip brasserie Balthazar in New York's Soho, where the signature salad has an ingredient for every letter in Balthazar including beets, asparagus, lettuces, truffle oil vinaigrette, haricots verts, avocado, lemon zest, anise (fennel), and radishes. Toss in one more player (at Balthazar they add some ricotta salata cheese) and you've got ten. As long as you've got the grill going . . . fire up dessert! Serve *grilled peach halves with low-fat vanilla frozen yogurt.* The contrast of hot and cold, caramelized and creamy, is delicious.

Okay, So These Are the Real Days of Our Lives

Some days you feel like eating carrots and some days it's got to be carrot cake. This we know. So, here are some strategies for dealing with the days when life gets in the way of a healthy lifestyle. The good news is that it can be done and research supports it. Dr. John Foreyt, director of the Behavioral Medicine Research Center at Baylor College of Medicine in Houston, says that the keys to long-term weight control are problem solving on a daily basis, predicting challenges, and then planning for them. "People may say they *want* a detailed prescribed meal plan, but what they *need* is nutrition know-how and the problem-solving skills to use any day of their lives." So, let's solve a few problems one day at a time!

> Tell me what you eat and I will tell you who you are.
> —Anthelme Brillat-Savarin, *The Physiology of Taste*, 1825

✳ For Those Days When It's the Food

"I don't feel like cooking." On those days when you're dog-tired and you just can't muster up the motivation to start whipping out those pots and pans, don't be shy about taking advantage of convenience foods and takeout. The sky's the limit these days, from frozen organic entrées and next-to-fresh pasta and sauces from the supermarket, to takeout fish tacos and grilled chicken salads from a nearby drive-thru. Just bear in mind a few tips before you zap that frozen dinner in the microwave or pull that takeout menu from the drawer. Think healthy. Just because you're taking a cooking shortcut doesn't mean you've

lowered your standards. Always keep a few frozen vegetables, entrées, or "meal makers," such as individually frozen chicken breasts, on hand. You never know which day is going to leave you hungry but unwilling to cook. Frozen entrées are good too. Just read the nutrition labels to pick the healthiest ones.

Stock up on frozen and canned veggies. Frozen broccoli spears or canned corn are better than no veggies at all. In fact, some frozen vegetables actually have more vitamins than their fresh counterparts.

If takeout is your way out, you're in luck because more restaurants than ever are geared up to offer their whole menu for the carry-out crowd. That means you can enjoy a well-balanced dinner at home and let someone else do the cooking.

Take advantage of the ever-growing selections of prepackaged salad fixin's. Some come with an impressive salad bar blend of lettuces, carrots, snow peas, and radishes. Just open the bag and serve with your favorite reduced-fat salad dressing or a little olive oil and balsamic vinegar.

Keep an eye on sodium. Convenience and fast foods are notorious for packing a big sodium wallop. Sodium won't make you fat, but could leave you feeling fatter.

"I've just got to have fries today." Eating healthy over the long run means there's room for splurge foods you crave on occasion. So when your taste buds crave French fries, order up! Obviously, a small order is the way to go to limit fat and calories. But there's something else at play here too. The nutrition impact of eating carbs like potatoes is influenced by what you eat *with* them. Potatoes rate pretty high on the glycemic index (GI) scale. That is the measure of a food's impact on how fast and high our blood sugar levels go after we eat it. The theory is that high GI foods (like white potatoes, pasta, white bread, rice, and sugar) cause a rapid rise in blood sugar. That prompts the pancreas to pump out insulin to lower blood sugar, which triggers a craving for another carbohydrate fix, leading to an endless cycle of carbo-crazy eating. But you can tighten security to slow the flow of insulin, because the

nutrition impact of eating simple carbs is influenced by what you eat *with* them. Dr. Dean Ornish, famous for his work on nutrition and reversal of heart disease, as the founder of the Preventive Medicine Research Institute at the University of California in San Francisco, explains, "While it is true that some foods such as potatoes have a high glycemic index, most people don't make a meal out of just one food. When eaten with other foods that are high in fiber and thus have a low glycemic index, such as whole grains and most vegetables, then the fiber in the other foods slows the rate of absorption of all of the foods eaten during that meal." So, eat your fries with a meal containing protein and preferably a salad filled with high-fiber veggies, and you're the boss controlling blood sugar's bouncing ball.

Suggested reading: Eat More, Weigh Less, Dr. Dean Ornish (Quill, 2001).

"I'm going to a big bash tonight." Cocktail-hour calories can really add up. So, why not get in the habit of adding a few "Mocktails" to the mix? Sure, you can enjoy a couple of glasses of white wine or cosmos with friends. But after that, order a club soda with a splash of cranberry juice or grapefruit juice and a twist of lime and you'll save at least 100 calories each time you make the substitution. You're also rehydrating so you'll look much more refreshed in the morning! (For more on mocktails, see chapter 6, The Dish on Drinks.)

"I'm not in the mood for a boring salad." Well, then don't make one! Get out of the lettuce and tomato rut and get creative. The recipe that follows is from Xavier and Nina Teixido, owners of Harry's Savoy Grill and Ballroom in Wilmington, Delaware. Xavier was the chairman of the National Restaurant Association in 2002, which required him to travel to just about all of the fifty states and eat out, of course! He joked, "I knew the year would be a personal success if at the end I still had a wife, still had a restaurant, and could still fit into my pants!" We asked him for his favorite salad recipe and he enthusiastically said, "It has to be the avocado-arugula salad with grapefruit vinaigrette!"

Avocado and Arugula with Grapefruit Vinaigrette

Xavier Teixido, owner and food lover, Harry's Savoy Grill and Ballroom, Wilmington, Delaware

YIELD: *4 servings*

For the salad:

1 to 2 heads Bibb lettuce, washed and patted dry

1 bunch arugulas

2 avocados, peeled and sliced lengthwise

2 grapefruit peeled and segmented, reserve excess juice

1 cup green grapes, seeded and halved, may be peeled

½ cup julienned red pepper

2 tablespoons minced fresh chives or Italian parsley

½ cup pecans or walnuts, toasted

For the dressing:

⅔ cup extra-virgin olive oil

⅓ cup sherry vinegar or red wine vinegar

1 tablespoon reserved fresh grapefruit juice

Kosher salt and black pepper to taste

1   On four chilled plates equally divide the Bibb and arugula.

2   On the bed of greens, arrange the avocado slices and grapefruit segments.

3   Garnish with the grapes and red pepper.

4   Combine the ingredients for the dressing and drizzle over the entire salad.

5   Add a final garnish of the minced chives or parsley and the toasted nuts. Serve chilled.

Xavier suggests: Sauvignon Blanc, Pinot Gris, or dry Reisling.

"I scream for ice cream today." Okay, you've got two choices here. Choose a lower-fat frozen dairy dessert that still delivers the creamy deliciousness you crave without as many calories. Or get real with real ice cream and scoop wisely. Unless you want your pants to split, skip the five-hundred-calories-and-up banana split with three or four scoops of ice cream, plus bananas, nuts, chocolate sauce, and whipped cream. And note that ice cream brands vary wildly in fat content. A half cup of don't-wear-a-bikini-with-this-one Macadamia Brittle Häagen-Dazs sports 26 grams of fat and 360 calories, while the same serving size of Breyers All Natural Vanilla ice cream has a more acceptable 8 grams of fat and 140 calories. Throw some fresh strawberries or blueberries on top to make your frozen dream even happier.

FYI: Another taste option that may quiet down that primal ice cream scream is frozen yogurt, like TCBY's reduced-fat (96% fat-free) frozen yogurt, which clocks in at 140 calories and 3 grams of fat per half-cup serving. No more calorie savings, but less fat.

"I want to eat popcorn at the movies today." Dinner and a movie? Believe it or don't, a tub of popcorn with a soft drink can rack up more calories than the meal you just had. Here's what to do. You be the director and make a decision on what to cut. Dessert at dinner or popcorn at the movie? There's just no room for double billing here. Can't make it through the movie without popcorn? Get the smallest tub available and split it. Some theaters offer kids' tubs. Still bigger than the official three-cup serving, but it's the smallest container you can buy. And just say "No" to the yellow grease they pour on top. Avoid sugary soft drinks. Even the "smalls" are gargantuan. Order bottled water instead or let this be your diet-drink occasion. Munch slowly and make it last. If you scarf down the popcorn before the previews are even over, you'll be diving into your movie mate's popcorn tub before you can say, "Action!"

"*Nothing tastes good to me today.*" It's all about finding flavor, and the search for something that tastes good is a powerful one. After all, the European quest for spices launched the age of explorers. "Wake up your taste buds" is a common expression and sensory science researchers tell us it really involves our noses too. So, the aromas of foods cooking can get our taste buds going again. Actually, it's really the brain that's the ultimate flavor finder. With every whiff or morsel, more than five million sensory cells swing into action. Combine that with the senses that detect color, texture, temperature, and even the sound of food (crunch!) and the brain creates the big picture that we call *flavor*. Here's a recipe for Southwest-Spiced Pork Tenderloin that's sure to liven things up with its salty, sweet, aromatic, hot, and spicy rub.

Southwest-Spiced Pork Tenderloin

From the creative minds and kitchens of the *National Pork Board*

YIELD: *4 servings*

1 tablespoon paprika

1½ teaspoons salt

1½ teaspoons brown sugar

1½ teaspoons granulated sugar

1½ teaspoons chili powder

1½ teaspoons ground cumin

1½ teaspoons black pepper

1 whole pork tenderloin, about 1 pound

1. In small bowl, stir together the paprika, salt, brown sugar, granulated sugar, chili powder, ground cumin, and black pepper until thoroughly blended. (Makes ¼ cup.)

2. Heat the oven to 425 degrees F. Season the tenderloin with 2 tablespoons of the rub. Place the tenderloin in a shallow pan and roast for 30 to 35 minutes, until the internal temperature as measured with a meat or instant-read thermometer is 155 degrees F.

3. Remove the pork from the oven and let rest 5 minutes. Slice the tenderloin and serve.

✳ It's the Way You Feel Today

"My jeans feel too tight today and I want to fit into my little black dress tomorrow night!" You know it's impossible to knock off a few pounds of body fat in one day, but if bloating is causing that too-fat-to-fit feeling, there are a few steps you can take today to help you slide into that little black number tomorrow—without resorting to control top pantyhose. Do the regular healthy thing, eat lots of *fruits* and *vegetables* and drink lots and lots of *water*. The more you drink, the more relief you'll get from temporary bloating. Constipated? Think E's and F's. Exercise and fiber. Exercise and eat a high-fiber diet today and you may get relief in time for tomorrow night. Put *grapefruit juice* on the menu. It has natural diuretic properties that help to flush out all that fluid that's making you feel so fat. And go easy on the salt. Nothing can make you puff up faster than salty snacks and a day's menu of salty, processed foods. Oh, and save the alcohol for tomorrow night. Partaking tonight could mean puffing up tomorrow.

"I'm having a bad day and deserve to splurge." Could it *be* any worse? Well, yeah, it could, if you decide to go hog wild and eat all of tomorrow's calories today. That's not exactly the formula for a brighter day. Don't let your emotions get the best of you. A little splurge, you deserve. Anything more is an exercise in masochistic overeating. Try this on for size: Make a list of your favorite comfort foods—cream-filled chocolates, strawberry milk shake, mint Milano cookies, tiramisu-flavored ice cream—and decide on an acceptable "splurge"-sized serving. When you sense that urge to splurge coming on, check out your list and do your best to stick with those less-damaging servings. Dr. John Foreyt, of the Baylor College of Medicine, says it's a matter of minimizing the damage done. Don't put your emotions in the driver's seat. You're the one in control of how you feel and what you eat. What's that? You feel like self-control and splurging are mutually exclusive terms? Then just be prepared to pay the piper for the next several days with extra activity and a little trimming here and there on calories.

"I made it to the gym this morning and I want to keep that powerful feeling going." You're definitely starting off on the right foot. Just the fact that you've already gotten up and gotten moving puts the odds in your favor that this is going to be a good nutrition day. There's nothing like starting off the day with a workout, a jog, or a power walk to put you in the right frame of mind for healthy eating. Dr. Foreyt says it best: "Exercise improves well-being and people who feel good are in better control of their diets and their lives." Still, it doesn't hurt to make that extra effort to focus on high-energy foods that don't leave you feeling dragged down. Because motivation is high, the days you work out are the best time to try to make up for that lemon cheesecake splurge earlier in the week. Focus on complex carbs, like whole-grain cereals, breads, and crackers; go easy on the fat and fill up on lots of fresh fruit. And be sure to get plenty of water throughout the day. Chances are you lost more than you realize with your workout.

"I stepped on the scale this morning and lo and behold, I lost two pounds. I feel like I'm on the right track and I don't want to veer off." Like exercise, weight loss is motivating. Just don't go overboard and try to starve yourself today in an effort to speed things up a bit. The best way to parlay that two-pound loss into a three-pound loss, or more, is to keep doing what you're doing. That's not to say you can't shave off another hundred calories, if things have been going well and you haven't felt deprived. But choose your calorie-cuts wisely. The best calories to say *arrivederci* to are the ones in those high-fat, high-sugar, low-nutrient splurges that you so adore. If doing without is going to lead to crazy cravings, then why fix what ain't broke? Just be patient and the other pounds will follow.

✳ It's Your Schedule Today

"I have to drive in the car for like three or four hours today." Road trip! Keeping a small cooler filled with survival snacks such as bottled water, baby carrots, drinkable yogurts, and fresh fruit outfits the ultimate driving machine. Light snacks and staying hydrated is good to keep you alert. But avoid munching out of boredom. You could fall victim to a hundred miles of mindless corn-chip consumption. Whether for work or the weekend, a long car ride often means stopping at convenience stores for refueling you and your car. Happily, there have been a few highway improvements in the snack lane. There's a lot more than beef jerky and big gulps to choose from now, so there's no excuse to overfill *your* tank. Instead, pick some high-performance fuels such as citrus juices, packets of nuts, oatmeal snack bars, or a carton of low-fat milk. More convenience store chains are working to broaden their choices with health-minded road warriors in mind. As Jim Keyes, President of 7-Eleven points out, "Drinks have to fit in a car-cup holder. Square orange juice cartons can't do that. That's why we like Tropicana's new single serving plastic bottles. It's OJ to go." Do we get a car wash with that?

Hawaiian Health and Bounty

Going on vacation doesn't have to mean leaving fitness goals at home anymore. So the pressure is on for hotel and resort chefs. It's not always a day at the beach when they have to please guests who not only want to look great in their bathing suits, they actually eat in their bathing suits lounging by the pool. So, Kurt Matsumoto, managing director of Mauna Lani Bay Hotel and Spa on the big island of Hawaii, makes sure guests surfing their menus will find lots of light dishes featuring local fresh fish and tropical produce. It also means making sure his wait staff is as experienced with the menu as the cabana boys are with rescuing you from a runaway catamaran. "Help! What should I order!"

"People are more educated and eating differently, so our chefs and waiters have to be more educated. These are active vacationers who snorkel, play golf, hike, and kayak." Then it's off to the body-baring spa! Add the influence of Asian cuisine to Hawaii's fresh ingredients and it can be ono-licious. (Ono is Hawaiian for delicious!)

Carolyn Says: One of my favorite dishes enjoyed at the Mauna Lani Bay Terrace, while evening breezes rustled in the palms, is Opakapaka (pink snapper) in a ginger broth with Asian vegetables.

Braised Opakapaka in Ginger and Exotic Mushroom Broth

Edwin Goto, Executive Chef, Mauna Lani Bay Hotel, Hawaii

YIELD: *5 servings*

For fish:

Five 5-ounce portions Opakapaka or firm white fish (bass, snapper, grouper), seasoned with salt

1 recipe ginger broth (below)

4 cups sliced mushrooms, assorted variety of shiitake, oyster, or button mushrooms (save stems for broth)

½ cup chopped green onions

Kosher salt to taste

Freshly ground black pepper to taste

Lemon juice to taste

½ cup ginger, julienned

½ cup carrots, diced

1 Preheat the oven to 350 degrees F. Make ginger broth (see below).

2 Transfer the ginger broth to a casserole dish with a fitted cover large enough to hold five portions of Opakapaka. Add the mushrooms and fish.

3 Place in the oven and cook covered for 12 to 15 minutes, or until done. (Cooking time will vary by the thickness of the fish.)

4 Remove the casserole from the oven and transfer the fish to serving bowls. Taste the broth and adjust the flavor with lemon juice, salt, and freshly ground pepper.

5 Ladle the broth and the mushrooms over the fish. Garnish with sliced green onions, julienned ginger, and small diced and blanched carrots. Serve immediately.

For broth:

Ginger broth can be made a day ahead

1 quart water

1 cup dry white wine

1 small carrot, diced

1 stalk celery, diced

1 5-inch piece of ginger, diced into ¼-inch pieces

2 cloves garlic, crushed

1 small onion, peeled and diced

1 green onion, minced

1 sprig Italian parsley, stems only

1 sprig fresh thyme

1 bay leaf

Stems and trimmings from mushrooms used for the fish

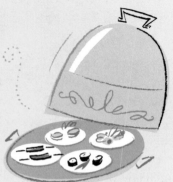

1 In a saucepot combine the water and white wine, bring to a boil, and then simmer over low heat for 5 minutes.

2 Add the remaining ingredients and allow broth to simmer for an additional 20 minutes.

3 Cool broth. Strain through a fine mesh strainer and store in the refrigerator until ready to use.

Fish can be served with steamed Jasmine rice on the side, and green Asian vegetables such as baby bok choy, snow peas, or choi sum (Chinese broccoli).

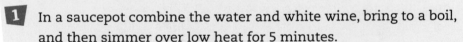

Hip & Healthy Heroine: Rhonda Rowland

"I'm on the Road Eating Lunch with Coworkers Today."

For real-life advice on this one we go live to ask former CNN Medical Correspondent Rhonda Rowland how she avoided the extra pounds while pounding the pavement nationwide gathering the latest medical news. "It was always a challenge to get lunch in. Also, all that adrenaline gets you to burn off food quickly. On the road—while we know many reporters would take the crews to fast-food restaurants, I always made sure we carved out time to eat at a restaurant, or at a hospital cafeteria if that wasn't an option. Being on the road was not an excuse to eat burgers and fries (though many of our crews did!) or splurge on dessert. If possible, I'd pick out a Chinese or Thai restaurant since you can always eat low-fat. I stuck to my guns about ordering chicken, pasta, or salads in restaurants. At night, same thing—I often ordered fish or pasta. But I was always concerned about picking up extra pounds on the road." BTW: She didn't!

"I have to sit on an airplane for hours." This is bound to be a day where you don't get the physical exercise you need but your nerves will sure get a workout! Get ready for the glamour of modern-day travel—standing in security lines, waiting for delayed flights, jostling with fellow passengers to store your carry-on, sitting on the runway, accepting an airline snack mix, and eventually making it to your destination. Since airline meals are disappearing too, here are a few travel-tested tips to help you navigate nutritiously when you fly.

Start the day ready for battle with a good breakfast including fiber-rich and filling whole-grain cereal or oatmeal and a big glass of orange juice. The hundreds of nutrients in OJ help boost your immune system to give you a fighting chance to ward off cold and flu germs floating in the cabin air on crowded flights.

Make your own Sky Trail Mix comprised of peanuts, almonds, raisins, and other dried fruits. Healthy fats and stomach-filling fiber will keep you going and this combo will be much lower in sodium than the on-board snack mixes. You want to cut down on sodium intake today, because all that sitting can lead to unwanted puffiness and even ankle swelling. So, make sure to ask yourself if you are really famished. The good news is that most airports do have healthier choices today. Used to be the only thing you could get was a hot dog and soda; now many airports have outlets selling freshly made sandwiches, salads, yogurts, and even sushi. A salad is fine, but make sure it contains some kind of protein, such as chicken, turkey, ham, eggs, or cheese, to keep your blood sugar on an even keel. Stress can take a toll, driving your blood sugar level down way below normal.

Be sure to stay hydrated. Another reason to carry your own bottled water—chances are you'll be beyond thirsty by the time the flight attendant drink cart reaches your row. Which brings us to alcohol at altitude. Skip the wine and drink the water. You and your skin and your brain can really get dehydrated in a pressurized cabin. If it's at the end of a long travel day and you want a drink to unwind, that's fine. But make sure to double up on water with the wine.

If you happen to be on one of the last remaining flights on the planet that serves a meal, know that you can order a special one ahead of time. Airlines request a minimum of twenty-four-hours notice. Special meals usually include fruit for dessert, which is much better than the glue-like cube that passes for cake served with regular meals. But if you do have a regular meal, we recommend you eat the main dish, the salad, half the bread, and offer the dessert to the guy sitting next to you. He looks hungry.

Hip & Healthy Heroine:
Anita Cotter

"I'm Staying in a Hotel Today."

Traveling for your job sounds so glamorous, but it can become a problem when it's not your suitcase that's getting heavier! Our travel pro friend Anita Cotter, Director of Public Relations, the Americas for the Savoy Hotel Group, knows this challenge well. Anita lives in New York to promote the Savoy Group, but all of the hotels she represents are in London, so she is truly a jet-setter "crossing the pond" several times a year. So here's Anita on *healthy hotel living*. "My schedule can be exhausting when I travel. I find a thirty-minute workout at the end of the day before dinner can be a wonderful energizer. It's better than a nap and it burns some calories. I try to schedule the time when I plan my itinerary, because I feel better when I'm in important meetings."

Happily, fitness centers and spas are standard equipment at most major hotels these days. "Guests simply demand a good workout facility. If a particular hotel doesn't have workout options, shop around for one that does. Many hotels, such as the Berkeley and the Savoy in the heart of London, have pools along with extensive weight-training equipment." Anita points out that if you like to go exploring while you exercise, many hotels also provide jogging maps with safe routes in the area of the hotel. "And the hotel staff can often arrange for a running mate if you're nervous about being alone."

And since part of the fun of traveling is enjoying the food, Anita has some gourmet goals as well. "On my London trips, if I know I'm dining at, say, Gordon Ramsay's restaurant at Claridge's on a particular night, I'll save my calories for the wonderful experience and go light at breakfast and lunch." But, she says, beware of the room service continental breakfast pastry basket. "There's enough in there for a week. I try to order an English muffin or cereal with skim milk instead." As hard as you try, it's easy to gain a few pounds on a trip. But Anita has a plan for that too. "If I cut back right away when I get home, the pounds tend to disappear quickly. My clothes usually tell me everything I need to know!" Anita, daahling, you look fabulous!

✳ It's Not Me Today

"I was going to eat a salad at my desk, but now I've been invited out to lunch." **Salad solution #1:** Flexibility is the key to success. It's all about choices, remember? The simplest solution is to have that salad for dinner. If it deteriorates into a wilted mess by dinnertime, then toss it and make another. Or stop by a deli or other salad bar to-go eatery for a made-to-order salad on your way home. What should you put in the salad? Your choices are limited only by the salad bar selections and your degree of indulgence at the noon meal. And don't forget that salad bars can offer some pretty hefty, high-calorie items too, like macaroni salad, bacon, grated cheese, potato salad, coleslaw, and tons o' dressing. Choose wisely. Size matters.

Salad solution #2: Eat the salad before you go to lunch. Pennsylvania State University researchers found that dieters who start their lunch with a big but low-calorie salad end up eating less total calories. Nutrition professor Barbara Rolls Ph.D., author of *The Volumetrics Weight-Control Plan* (Quill, 2000), says that larger salads were better than smaller ones at shaving calories from the meal. Eating three cups of low-fat salad resulted in a 12 percent overall reduction in lunch calories compared with 7 percent fewer calories for those who ate 1½ cups of salad. Apparently, time-tested advice to "fill up on salad first" is now research proven. And it turns out the study also shows that dieters felt just as full on three cups of salad, whether it contained one hundred or four hundred calories. So, no need to pour on the dressing. Another example of the more you know, the more you can eat!

"I didn't pick this restaurant!" Hey, bummer, you're not always in charge. And sometimes you've got to go with the gang on a restaurant ride to a place that you'd normally drive right by. Now, before they ask you, "Would you like some cheese with that whine?" sharpen your menu-reading skills and open your mind to find a real meal. You can always shout, "I'm allergic to fried clam strips!" to avoid the deep-fried shared appetizer blitz or suggest the buffalo chicken wings that come with celery sticks and nibble on more of those than the fried bird. Then choose your own entrée à la Meg

Ryan in *When Harry Met Sally* and get to work ordering this or that on the side, with or without these or those until you're happy with your cuisine and its calorie count. Hey, you're smiling again. I'll have what she's having!

"My guy loves lasagna so I'm making that for dinner." Okay, sometimes love makes us do things we don't want to do. And since, as the saying goes, the way to a man's heart is through his stomach, the recipe for catch-a-man stew is often a little more rib sticking than the way we gals normally eat. There are two approaches here. **One:** You join in the food fun and make whatever he loves and just cut back during the day to prepare for the food of love. (*You* know how to do that!) Or, **Two:** You find a bet-ya-can't-tell recipe that serves up full-boat flavors without all the full-fat calories. A great resource for recipes with makeovers is *www.cookinglight.com*. As the website for *Cooking Light* magazine, you'll hit the recipe jackpot, once you log on.

Let's Get Personal

The personal touch matters. Whether it's choosing a hair stylist or a decorator, you want a professional who listens to your unique needs and tastes. The same goes when looking for nutrition advice. If you're serious about making some specific and long-term changes in the way you eat and want the best results, then go to *the* nutrition expert—a registered dietitian. RDs can be found in the yellow pages or you can ask your doctor for a referral. Or you can log on to *www.eatright.org* to find a dietitian in your area.

They usually charge by the hour and range from $75 to $100 a visit. But, hey! That's less than hair highlights and less than most decorators, so get your priorities straight. You're worth it! Sometimes nutrition counseling is covered by health insurance plans, sometimes it's not. So, check on that too. What you get is a diet tailored to your lifestyle. When you're really in a bind, grab the cell and call your dietitian! "Help! I can't decide between the Southwestern Chicken Chile or the Beef Fajitas!"

FINAL THOUGHTS on Eating Healthy and Being Fabulous!

If you're sneaking ahead and reading this first, here's what the book's about. Or maybe you're actually reading it last. Here's where we've been: Nutrition is not a long list of all of the things you cannot eat. Instead choose the foods that give you life, energy, and health. Accessorize sensibly with high-fat and sugary treats. Eat the foods you love and learn to love the foods you need for good health. Take some cooking classes. Go out and play and get physical every day, even if it's taking the stairs one day and climbing a mountain the next. Stand up straight and laugh with your friends. Take a multivitamin, because nobody's perfect. Taste something new. Use this book to find nutrition facts and fantastic foods, because the more you know, the more you can eat. Now, that's fabulous!

Your Dish Divas,

Carolyn and Densie
www.dishdivas.com

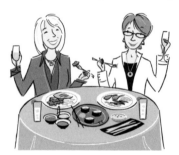

Index

counting of, 37–40, 275–76
cutting of, 35, 38–39, 85,
	275–76
in dairy products, 129–30, 131,
	132–33, 341
meal plans low in, 330–37
in nonalcoholic drinks, 201,
	206, 217, 219
in oil, 71
in party snacks, 245
in restaurant items, 169, 174,
	176, 188, 189
in spreads, 132–33, 174
see also exercise
Campos, Eremita, 142
cancer, 49, 53, 55, 59, 66, 70, 73,
	77, 81, 82, 84, 86, 87, 88, 89,
	90, 95, 211
see also specific cancers
cantaloupe, 82
carbohydrates, 37, 42–44, 71, 320,
	331
complex, 42–43, 344
cravings for, 274–77, 283
diets low in, 42
fats vs., 45
nutrition impact of, 338–39
carrot juice, 207
carrots, 82, 138
Centers for Disease Control and
	Prevention, 147, 289, 290,
	293, 298
cereals, 74, 75, 92–93, 327
fiber content in, 17, 114
shelf life of, 108
see also whole grains

Cetaphil Lotion, 313
champagne, 223–24, 230
	"pink," 225–26
Champagne Veuve Clicquot, 224
Chanel, Coco, 184
Chappellet, Molly, 255
cheating, 9, 269–85
appetite vs. hunger in, 282–83
diet support Web sites on, 285
minimizing damage of,
	275–79, 338–39, 341, 344
tips on, 283–85
on weekends, 282
see also cravings; triggers,
	eating
cheese, 74, 129–30, 327
mold on, 130
shelf life of, 150
see also dairy
cheesecake:
banana split, 278–79
reduced fat, 276–79
Cheesecake Factory, The, 187
cheese grater, 104
cherries, 83
chestnuts, 69
Chez Panisse, 91
chicken breasts:
accessorizing of, 159
green chile, 161
lemon caper, 160
sauté, 160
taste of Thai chicken, 161
tomato garlic, 161
see also poultry
Child, Julia, 151–52, 220, 239–40

117, 140, 148, 205, 211, 327, 331, 349, 350
two types of, 54
fidgeting, 21, 308
fines-herbes, classic omelet, 136–37
fish, 74, 84, 315, 331
  canned, 147
  cooking of, 157
  healthiest choices in, 146–48
  shelf life of, 150
  omega-3 content of, 98–99
  see also seafood
fitness, *see* exercise
flaxseed, 84, 98, 315
Fleming, Claudia, 267
Floataway Café, 247
folate, 88, 89, 229
Fonda, Jane, 305
food:
  clearing pantry of, 105–8
  condiments for, 148–49
  cooking of, 151–61
  frozen, 149–50
  shelf life of, 107–8
  stocking up on, 127–51
  see also diets, dieting; nutrition; *specific foods*
Food and Drug Administration (FDA), 86–87, 98, 111, 147
Food and Nutrition Board of the National Academy of Sciences, 41, 326
Food & Wine Magazine Classic, The, 221, 256
food journals, 6, 275

Food Lover's Companion (Herbst), 172
food processor, 103
Foreyt, John, 294, 337, 344
fortified juice, 93
Franklin, Benjamin, 225
frozen dinners, 56, 149–50, 338
fruit crisp, 262
fruits, 60–62, 331, 343, 344
  canned, 118–19
  color in, 64, 197
  daily servings of, 62, 327
  in desserts, 266, 331
  juice vs. whole, 205
  shelf life of, 138–39
  serving sizes of, 328
  smoothies, 219
  as source of water, 73, 74
  see also produce; *specific fruits*
frying, 158–59

garlic, tomato chicken, 161
garlic press, 104
Gatorade Sports Institute, 302
Georgia, Medical College of, 317
Georgia Campaign for Adolescent Pregnancy Prevention (G-CAPP), 305
Gift of Southern Cooking, The (Peacock and Lewis), 152
Gilbert, Linda, 168–69
ginger ale, homemade, 257
ginger and exotic mushroom broth, braised Opakapaka in, 347–48
glutathione, 79, 81

Splenda, 111, 204
spoons, measuring, 105
sports drinks, 217–18
spreads, 132–33, 331
    shelf life of, 150
starvation diets, x–ix
steak houses, 189
steamer, bamboo basket, 103
steaming, 156
Sterling, Joy, 244
stevia, 112
stewing, *see* braised, braising
stir-frying, 157
strawberries, 89, 139
Subway, 187
sucralose, 111, 204
sugar, 17, 43
    added, 43–44
    imitations of, 110–12, 204–5
    shelf life of, 108
    types of, 108–9
sunshine punch, 234
Superfoods, 77–99
    man-made, 92–95
    myths vs. facts on, 80–91
supplements, 52, 64
    energy bars as, 94
    selecting of, 74–75, 95–96, 98
    specialized, 96–97
    vitamin, 50, 51, 354
sushi, 147–48
Sweet'n Low, 111, 204

tae kwon do, 301
Tante Marie's Cooking School,
    159, 160

target heart rates, 299
taste of Thai chicken, 161
teas, 31, 66–67, 73, 74, 112–13,
    211–14
    bottled, 128–29
    caffeine content of, 67, 336
    fortified, 93
    health benefits of, 66, 89
    iced, 212, 213
    instant, 112
    shelf life of, 108
    sweetened, 44
    see also green tea
Teixido, Nina, 339
Teixido, Xavier, 339, 340
television, as eating trigger, 10–11
tenderloin:
    roasted beef, 262
    southwest-spiced pork, 342–43
TGI Friday's, 186
Thai chicken, taste of, 161
tofu, 41
tomatoes, 90, 139
tomato garlic chicken, 161
tomato juice, 206
tongs, 104
trainers, personal, 296–97, 309
trans fats, 43, 49, 119, 131
traveling, healthy eating in,
    28–31, 345–46, 349–51
Trefethen, Janet, 258, 259
triggers, eating, 4, 5–31, 34, 270,
    280–81
    carbs as, 338–39
    emotional, 8–9, 272–73
    identifying of, 5–31, 275